Aggressive Introvert

Aggressive Introvert

A STUDY OF HERBERT HOOVER

AND PUBLIC RELATIONS MANAGEMENT

1912–1932

CRAIG LLOYD

OHIO STATE UNIVERSITY PRESS : COLUMBUS : 1972

Library of Congress Cataloging in Publication Data

Lloyd, Craig.
  Aggressive introvert.

  Bibliography: p.
  1. Hoover, Herbert Clark, Pres. U.S., 1874-1964.
I. Title.
E802.L6   973.91'6'0924 [B]   72-12608
ISBN 0-8142-0181-4

To Caryl, my parents,
and the Donnelly's crowd

Contents

Preface

This work began as a project aimed at tracing the evolution of Herbert Hoover's social thought through his long public career. However, the realization that Hoover's thinking about society changed very little after 1920 and that a more useful study lay in an exploration of his administrative style led me to undertake the work that follows. For many people today, untouched by the Hoover rehabilitation that began in the late 1940s, the name Herbert Hoover still evokes a mental image of bungling incompetence—though among the young this image is perhaps more comic in its overtones than that which lingers in the minds of those who remember the depression. If the wry expressions I received from fellow students and colleagues upon learning of the subject of my research are any indication, the under-thirty generation has a tendency to dismiss Hoover as a hapless simpleton who was once fittingly introduced before a national radio audience as "Hoobert Hevert." At the very least, I hope that my examination of Hoover's personality and its relationship to his administrative style will serve as a corrective to the distorted images of a man who was deeply committed to finding solutions to the problems confronting modern America. I do not mean my book to be a "brief" for either Hoover or his policies; but in an age of unmanageable and impersonal bureaucracies and all too consciously contrived "high" and "low profile" presidents, it is a grave injustice to continue to regard the personality and political style of Herbert Hoover as a species of historical comedy.

Many individuals assisted me in the research and writing which went into the preparation of this book. First and foremost, Ellis W. Hawley of the University of Iowa read the manuscript with great care and offered innumerable suggestions for improving the text.

I wish to extend to him my heartfelt appreciation for his helpfulness. Thanks also are due to David Burner of the State University of New York at Stony Brook, who raised a number of helpful questions and who graciously made available to me some of his own research materials. Robert R. Dykstra of the University of Iowa provided great assistance when the project was in its early stages, and Christopher Lasch of the University of Rochester, though not involved in my Hoover work, gave me invaluable instruction and stimulation in historical inquiry and therefore deserves mention as an indirect contributor to this work. Needless to say, the conclusions that I have drawn and any errors that may exist in the text are entirely my own.

Without the aid of a Teaching-Research Fellowship granted me by the Graduate Faculty of the University of Iowa, the undertaking of this work would have been difficult indeed. Then, too, the members of the staff of the Herbert Hoover Presidential Library, especially, former Acting Director Richard A. Jacobs, Director Thomas T. Thalken, Assistant Director Robert W. Woods, Archivists Dwight M. Miller and Mrs. Trudy Peterson, Librarian Mrs. Ruth Dennis, and special assistant Mrs. Mildred Mather, were always extremely cooperative and greatly facilitated the process of research. To them and to Miss Ada Stoflet of the University of Iowa library staff, I am deeply indebted. I am grateful as well for the skilled editorial work of Robert S. Demorest and the other staff members of the Ohio State University Press.

Finally, I must thank my wife, Caryl A. Lefstad Lloyd, for her unfailing encouragement.

Introduction

This study seeks to fill a gap in the existing historical literature about Herbert Hoover by providing a thematic analysis of one major facet of his life and career, namely, his development and use of an administrative style that relied heavily upon public relations techniques and was closely tied to a complex personality and deeply held philosophical commitments. To date, studies of this sort have been rare. Instead, the bulk of research and writing on Hoover has tended to consist either of unsystematic, journalistic biographies marked (and often marred) by strong biases pro and con, or, more recently, scholarly works dealing with quite specific phases or aspects of his career.[1]

That no disciplined, wide-ranging studies have appeared in the almost four decades since Hoover left the White House is perhaps best explained in terms of the unique nature of his career and personality. The former, rising swiftly as it did, out of orphanage, obscurity, and poverty in the American West to international wealth, esteem, and influence and ultimately on to the American presidency, was truly epic. Its sheer scope and variety, combined until recently with the unavailability of primary research materials,[2] have made treatment of it difficult and have thus far permitted only the most cursory description. Similarly, the puzzling personality of the man—of an individual who was at once a blend of small town American Quaker, professional mining engineer and scientist, and cosmopolitan administrator of huge organizations the world over—has made the search for meaningful continuity a difficult one, particularly since Hoover's was a personality that cherished privacy and habitually sought concealment. This desire to shroud all matters pertaining to his private life was a trait that plagued his interviewers, biographers, and aides throughout his career,[3] and one that left his own writings almost totally devoid of the kind of personal commentary that would be helpful to the historian in accounting for his remarkable achievement and ultimate failure. For him, the only things worth recording about his life were his "accomplishments," which he once defined as "the origination or administration of tangible institutions or constructive works." "Conversation and gossip" and descriptions of personal life not related to accomplishment were "useless adornments" and "therefore omitted" from his narrative.[4]

Ironically, it has been in Hoover's very tendency to guard his privacy and in his strong need to avoid public exposure that I have found the major analytical theme that underlies my inquiry. For materials in the Herbert Hoover Presidential Library and the Hoover Institution on War, Revolution, and Peace, together with evidence in his own published writings, in the articles and biographies written by his close friends, and in the autobiographies of his associates, suggest that Hoover developed what I shall refer to as a "behind-the-scenes, public relations" administrative approach, primarily to suit the needs of his outstanding personality trait, his tendency to shrink before the public eye. Using the press and public relations to a degree extraordinary for his times and habitually working through committees and conferences, he sought, as I shall try to demonstrate, to "reach out to the public" from behind the scenes, and by doing so, to win support for and implement the diverse programs and policies with which he was associated as chairman of the Commission for Relief in Belgium, food administrator, secretary of commerce, and president. Although shaped by personality factors, his commitment to this unique administrative style, I shall also argue, was strengthened by the political philosophy he formulated in the immediate post-World War I period.

This book, then, though more inclusive in scope than most scholarly works on Hoover, does not aim at anything approaching "definitive biography." At the descriptive level, it is concerned with documenting Hoover's studied mobilization of the press and public relations and with identifying the publicists, press agents, and public relations aides whom he brought into his service during his career. At the analytical level, it seeks to account for the formation of his complex personality and the idiosyncratic administrative style that grew out of it; to explain how his social outlook and political philosophy reinforced his commitment to this administrative style; to evaluate the charge leveled against him (a charge stemming from his employment of press agents) that he was using publicity to serve deep-seated presidential ambitions;[5] and, finally, to give a fuller understanding of his precipitous fall from public esteem between 1928 and 1932. Hopefully, through such description and analysis, the blurred historical focus on this largely still "unknown," but highly significant, American leader will have been sharpened.

1.   The journalistic biographies conveniently subdivide into three groups:

(1) Pre-presidential works written by close friends and associates of Hoover, e.g., Vernon Kellogg, *Herbert Hoover: The Man and His Work*; William Hard, *Who's Hoover?*; and Will Irwin, *Herbert Hoover: A Reminiscent Biography*. These works are laudatory treatments designed to acquaint the public with Hoover's virtues in election years in which he was a candidate for the presidency. Hard and Irwin appear to have written their books for campaign purposes. Irwin, a Stanford student with Hoover, provides the most useful information pertaining to Hoover's pre-1914 career.

(2)"Smear" biographies written during Hoover's presidency that unsuccessfully attempt to validate old political charges against Hoover, i.e., that he was financially dishonest, "really" an Englishman, and Machiavellian politically. Along with the bitterness engendered by the depression, Hoover's characteristic tendency to keep private the details of his personal life and career may have unwittingly helped spawn such vitriolic polemics as Walter Liggett's, *The Rise of Herbert Hoover* (New York, 1932); John Hamill's, *The Strange Career of Mr. Hoover under Two Flags* (New York, 1931); James O'Brien's *Hoover's Millions and How He Made Them* (New York, 1932); and Clement Wood's, *Herbert Clark Hoover: An American Tragedy* (New York, 1932).

(3) Works such as Herbert Corey's *The Truth about Hoover*, Eugene Lyons's *Our Unknown Ex-President*, David Hinshaw's *Herbert Hoover: American Quaker*, and Harold Wolfe's *Herbert Hoover: Public Servant and Leader of the Loyal Opposition* (New York, 1956), which have attempted to repudiate the "smears" and reestablish the pre-1929 view of Hoover as a man of remarkable achievement and idealism.

Recently published scholarly treatments of Hoover such as Harris G. Warren's *Herbert Hoover and the Great Depression* and Albert U. Romasco's *The Poverty of Abundance: Hoover, the Nation, the Depression* have dealt primarily with his presidency. Recent monographs that have utilized the manuscripts in the Herbert Hoover Presidential Library are: Bruce Alan Lohof, "Hoover and the Mississippi Valley Flood of 1927: A Case Study of the Political Thought of Herbert Hoover" (Syracuse, N.Y., 1968); Joan H. Wilson, *American Business and Foreign Policy,*

1920-1933 (Lexington, Ky., 1971); Glenn A. Johnson, "Secretary of Commerce Herbert C. Hoover: The First Regulator of American Broadcasting, 1921-1928" (Iowa City, 1970).

2. The Herbert Hoover Presidential Library in West Branch, Iowa, was only opened as recently as May, 1966. What materials the library contains pertaining to Hoover's pre-1914 career, however, are still largely restricted.

3. The very titles of some of the older books and articles about Hoover indicate the problems this "elusive" subject once posed even for interpreters who knew him well: for instance, Hard's *Who's Hoover?* and Lyons's *Our Unknown Ex-President*; also, Henry F. Pringle's "Hoover: An Enigma Easily Misunderstood" and Ray T. Tucker's "Is Hoover Human?".

4. Hoover makes these statements in a handwritten and very fragmentary chronicle of his pre-1914 career that was probably composed sometime during World War I (Box 1-Q/279, Herbert Hoover Papers, Herbert Hoover Presidential Library [hereafter cited as HHP, HHPL]). The same statements, however, might well also apply to his three-volume *Memoirs*, the first volume of which he prefaces with the comment: "These *Memoirs* are not a diary but a topical relation of some events and incidents in a roughly chronological order" (Herbert Clark Hoover, *The Memoirs of Herbert Hoover, 1874-1920: The Years of Adventure*, 1:v). Basically, his *Memoirs*, like the biographies that preceded them, are a narration of "constructive works."

5. Alfred W. McCann, "The Hoover Food-Control Failure," and [Clinton W. Gilbert], *The Mirrors of Washington*, pp. 120-21. During Hoover's presidency, critics such as Walter Lippmann, Heywood Broun, Robert Herrick, Drew Pearson, and Robert Allen, in reviewing his career, charged that he had assembled a "publicity machine" for the express purpose of becoming president: Walter Lippmann, "The Peculiar Weakness of Mr. Hoover," Heywood Broun, "It Seems to Heywood Broun," Robert Herrick, "Our Super-Babbitt: A Recantation," [Drew Pearson and Robert Allen], *Washington Merry-Go-Round*, p. 77; Robert Allen, *Why Hoover Faces Defeat*, pp. 1-10. Their general feeling was expressed in a *Nation* editorial: "During the whole of his public life [Hoover] has shown an incorrigible tendency to substitute words for action, to become a hero by publicity, not by deeds. . . . Never has any other person had a personal publicity machine as powerful and effective as the one that made Herbert Hoover President of the United States" ("Bally-hoover," p. 560). In 1935, *Time* was still referring to an alleged "astute and spectacular publicity build-up" that began during World War I and "ended by making Herbert Hoover a World Name and 31st President of the United States" ("Political Notes: Presidential Prose," *Time*, p. 8).

Aggressive Introvert

1 Drive and Diffidence

THE STORY OF HERBERT HOOVER'S RISE from the status of impoverished waif to multimillionaire, all within the space of three decades, makes the tales of Horatio Alger seem almost prosaic by comparison. And understandably, since these formative "years of adventure" have been obscured by his concern for privacy, they have lent themselves to myth-making and distortion on the part of his friends and enemies alike.[1] Fortunately, however, there are enough clues in Hoover's *Memoirs* and in the writings of his friends to give a fairly accurate accounting of the manner and methods of the man who emerged so suddenly onto the world stage in 1914. By assembling these clues, one can trace, in particular, the emergence of his behind-the-scenes style of action and his related interest in shaping public opinion via the press—both of which would later characterize his career in public administration.

I

Standard descriptions of Hoover's personality by writers and memoirists who had personal contact with him invariably make reference to his diffidence and reticence. The composite picture of Hoover formed by these accounts is that of a man who rarely looked directly at the person before him and who generally spoke only in terse replies to questions asked of him. Henry Pringle's 1928 description is representative of many accounts of Hoover's personality, a personality that—with respect to its outstanding

3

traits—does not seem to have altered much from adolescence to old age:

> He is abnormally shy, abnormally sensitive, filled with an impassioned pride in his personal integrity, and ever apprehensive that he may be made to appear ridiculous. . . . He rises awkwardly as a visitor is shown to his desk, and extends his hand only halfway, in a hesitant fashion. His clasp is less than crushing. Then he sits down and waits for questions. His answers are given in a rapid, terse manner and when he is finished he simply stops. Other men would look up, smile, or round off a phrase. Hoover is like a machine that has run down. Another question starts him off again. He stares at his shoes, and because he looks down so much of the time, the casual guest obtains only a hazy impression of his appearance.[2]

An analysis of the formation of Hoover's peculiar administrative style must begin by explaining his great need for privacy and the associated, much-celebrated personality traits—shyness and reticence—that Pringle describes so vividly. Although the very fact of this reticence makes accounting for it difficult, there are several factors in his youth that would seem to have some tangible bearing upon his character formation. To begin with, most biographers have seen his personal qualities as products, at least in some measure, of his rigorous Quaker upbringing. For instance, David Hinshaw, himself a Quaker and companion and aide to Hoover during his presidency, has written that "Quaker training and the inhibitions it creates" best account for his personality traits.[3] Eugene Lyons, relying primarily upon Hinshaw, argues in the same vein,[4] and such personal acquaintances of long standing as Will Irwin and William Hard also endeavor to relate Hoover's "repressed" personality to the austere discipline of his early environment.[5]

Such observations, moreover, though highly impressionistic, do appear to contain some validity. In works like Louis Thomas Jones's *The Quakers in Iowa*, one gets an insight into the strict discipline and character training that a frontier Quaker community such as West Branch, Iowa, Hoover's birthplace, imposed on its youth. The plain, unadorned homes and meeting house, the quiet piety and industry of the adults, the long silences of the

Quaker meeting itself, during which any youthful restlessness was punished—all of this created an atmosphere of restraint and simplicity of act and feeling, which would surely make itself felt upon anyone growing up within its confines.[6] Hoover himself, in one of his few statements about his Quaker youth, has written: "Those who are acquainted with the Quaker faith, and who know the primitive furnishing of the Quaker meeting-house, the solemnity of the long hours of meeting awaiting the spirit to move someone, will know the intense repression upon a ten-year-old boy who might not even count his toes."[7] In addition, one should not overlook the possible influence of the Quaker Queries, "the heart of Quaker discipline," which were read and answered monthly by regular attendants of the Quaker meetings. In part, Hoover's "personality style" may have been shaped by the moral precepts that the monthly recitation and answering of the Queries sought to internalize within the Quaker. In them, one could find strong strictures against "tale-bearing and detraction," strong disapproval of "involving [oneself] in business beyond [one's] ability to manage or in hazardous or speculative trade," and strong injunctions toward "plainness of speech, deportment, and apparel," "moderation and temperance on all occasions," and seeing to "the necessities of the poor,"[8] all of which may bear some relationship to Hoover's own personality and social attitudes. Such a code of behavior, after all, was the only socially acceptable one within the strict Quaker communities where he spent his first seventeen years. And he did remain a practicing Quaker throughout his life.

Along with the religious factor, it also seems plausible to relate Hoover's personality configuration to the emotional effects of his early orphanage and his youthful separation first from his brother and sister and then from his "second" family. His father died in 1880 when Hoover was only six years of age; his mother succumbed to pneumonia when he was nine.[9] These circumstances required that he part with his chief West Branch companions, his brother and sister, and that he go to live with the family of a paternal uncle on a farm near West Branch. Then, no sooner had he become a part of this "second" family than it was decided in intrafamily counsels that he should be sent to maternal relatives in

Newburg, Oregon. Hoover's mother had desired that her children receive a good education, and, since her brother, Dr. John Minthorn, was president of the Quaker academy in Newburg and himself recently bereft of a son, it was agreed that the boy be sent there. With characteristic unemotional terseness, Hoover, recalling this traumatic period of his life in his *Memoirs*, says simply, "In 1884 I was moved to Oregon."[10] Yet it seems justifiable to speculate with William Hard that his great need for a protective privacy, his "haltingness in manner towards people," "his most considerable personal inexpressiveness . . . was surely deepened by his early loss of the easy familiarities of home and his early subjection to the reticences and concealments inevitably induced by a life under alien roofs and in family circles related but strange."[11]

In 1891, Hoover, "a shy, repressed Quaker youth of seventeen," as he was remembered by contemporaries, entered Stanford University with its "Pioneer Class," the school having just been opened in the fall of that year. During his years with Dr. Minthorn, his main academic interests and successes had been in mathematics and his after-school work had been of an administrative nature, primarily as an assistant to Minthorn in the latter's newly founded land-settlement business. In addition, he deepened his interest in the operation and repair of machinery, something that can be traced as far back as the years on his uncle's farm in Iowa. Given these "leanings to the mechanical side," as he put it, he decided upon a career in engineering, made application to Stanford,[12] and although failing the English section of the entrance examination, was admitted conditionally on the basis of his evident determination and his ability in the mathematical subjects. Once in college, his deficiency in verbal expression continued to plague him. But he did well in his chosen specialties and managed to graduate when his geology and engineering professors succeeded in convincing the English Department that his ability to express himself in their areas was so great that he simply could not be denied the degree.[13]

While busy running a laundry service, delivering newspapers, and working as an assistant to his geology professor, Dr. John Branner, Hoover also found time to exercise and develop his administrative talents. Indeed, it seems likely that in the course of his Stanford career, he came to perceive that his way to prestige and influence lay in the carving-out of what might be called "an administrative sphere of competence." For Hoover, in spite of his shyness and inarticulateness, succeeded in becoming an important campus figure, chiefly by making himself and his administrative ability indispensable to the non-fraternity political faction, the "Barbarians" or "Barbs." Sharing their irritation over the fraternity group's monopolization of student government offices, its "favoritism in handling student enterprises and [its] loose methods of accounting for money," he suggested, in the course of dormitory "bull sessions," "a war for reform,"[14] especially for the adoption of a new constitution providing for more popular representation and insuring the honest handling of student funds. The proposal won the immediate approval of the "Barb" student leaders, and since no one else felt competent enough to administer it, Hoover himself agreed to run for treasurer on the "Barb" ticket, a campaign in which he was successful. Through the efforts of the more popular and politically oriented candidates, Lester Hinsdale and Herbert Hicks, the "3-H ticket" won the election and Hoover's reforms were instituted—reforms that remained a permanent part of Stanford student government and won the acclaim of Stanford's early presidents David Starr Jordan and Ray Lyman Wilbur.[15] Thus, at Stanford, one can note the initial emergence of what would later become Hoover's behind-the-scenes mode of administrative operation. Though too shy and inexpressive in public ever to be taken seriously as a bona fide leader himself, he had impressed the student leaders with the power and organizational cast of his mind;[16] and working through them, he was able to achieve influence and bring about action that he desired.

One might here make an instructive comparison of Woodrow Wilson's extracurricular collegiate activity with Hoover's. As Alexander George has recently pointed out, Wilson's constant writing and rewriting of student club constitutions at Johns Hopkins University was for him "a means of restructuring those institutional environments in which he wanted to exercise strong leadership by means of oratory, a skill in which he was adept as an adolescent and to the perfection of which he assiduously labored for years."[17] For Hoover, the reshaping of the Stanford student government constitution was a means by which he could develop and perfect his administrative aptitudes. Incapable of, and uninterested in, oratorical influence, Hoover devised a constitution that he could administer from the "unseen" office of the treasurer.

II

After graduating from Stanford University in 1895, Hoover embarked upon a career in mining engineering and administration, which would earn him a fortune of millions of dollars by 1914 and which carried him all over the globe.[18] In pursuit of this career, first as a member of the English mining firm, Bewick, Moreing and Company, and later on his own, he spent most of his time outside the United States, although after 1907 he did maintain offices in New York and San Francisco and kept close ties with Stanford and with Californian affairs generally. The key to his success lay partly in the excellent training in geological science that he had received from John Branner at Stanford, partly in his organizational and financial genius, particularly his ability to transform theretofore worthless mineral deposits and putatively exhausted mines into extremely valuable properties.[19] His base of operations after 1901 was London. Both his sons were born there; his rented home in Kensington, the Red House, was frequently visited by his many American and English friends and mining associates; and his sentimental, reminiscent attachment to the Red House suggests that if the Hoovers could be said to have had a home in the prewar years, it was London.[20] It was there, moreover, that his public career began. In the summer of 1914, while he was living at Red House and working on behalf of the San Francisco organizers of the Panama-Pacific Exposition, the war broke out. Germany invaded Belgium, and Hoover, after administering to the financial needs of stranded American tourists and expatriates, was sought out by influential American and Belgian businessmen to direct the administration of relief to the stricken Belgian people. With his acceptance, the end of his private career and start of his public one came about suddenly and in a manner totally unforeseen.

The accidental circumstances involved in Hoover's entry into public service, together with his striking personal diffidence and reticence, have tended to cast a legendary aura over the whole of his public career—the aura of the totally disinterested and "chaste" public servant who never derived any personal satisfaction whatever from his work. The biographies by Vernon Kellogg, William Hard, and David Hinshaw, for example, convey the impression that his entry into public life was both accidental and selfless, that he had never had any personal desire to be influential in the shaping of public policy, and that once involved, his ascent was not only purely fortuitous but also required continuous sacrifice in terms of wealth and personal comfort.[21] Hoover's own writings also contribute to this impression. In the preface to the second volume of his *Memoirs*, composed during his politically embittered post-presidential years, he wrote that only the desire "to ward off evils" threatening post-war America "caused me to spend practically all of the next fourteen years in public service; and I may remind doubting cynics that for money, mental satisfaction, physical comfort and reputation for myself and family, my profession was a far more enticing field."[22]

Hoover's *Memoirs* and some of his sympathetic biographers notwithstanding, it is hard to imagine any one entering and rising in government, whether it be at the local or national level, without having some motive beyond that of pure altruism. Surely a desire for prestige, for wielding influence, or for simply exercising one's talents in a new realm play a part in any man's decision to enter and remain in public life, and there is evidence that suggests Hoover was no exception here. David Starr Jordan, recalling a visit with the thirty-three year old Hoover in Australia in 1907, writes in his autobiography that even then Hoover was explaining "that he had run through his profession," that "it held nothing more for him, except to lay up money, of which he already had more than enough." He was planning to return to London, wind up his business affairs there, and then "go back to America and find some form of executive work in which he could be of service."[23] In 1910,

Jordan wrote to President William Howard Taft's secretary, apparently at the request of Hoover, calling attention "to a young man available for executive service," one, he said, who possessed "the greatest talent for work in that line," and was "very presentable . . . , of quiet, frank manner, but carrying conviction."[24] Hoover, the letter continued, "has risen to the front of his profession, having no superior in executive work, and have become [*sic*] a millionaire is now retiring at the age of 37 to return to America—probably to New York—with a view of entering public life." The letter brought him no position, but Hoover continued to think about one. In 1912, he was still complaining to Will Irwin, a Red House visitor at the time, that he was rich, "as rich as any man has a right to be," but "just money making wasn't enough." He was interested in getting "into the big game somewhere;" "interested in some job of public service—at home of course." When Irwin replied that it sounded as though Hoover was talking politics or government work, the latter remarked: "Well, I've always been interested in government and all that sort of thing; you remember Stanford. I don't know yet what it will be—but something."[25] Nor was Irwin the only one to whom he confided such sentiments. Mary Austin, another California writer and Hoover guest at the Red House, also remembers his lamenting that he "did not want to be just a rich man"; and she too was impressed with his interest in establishing "connections with his native land," an interest of which the United States "remained magnificently unaware."[26]

Contrary, then, to the impression that Hoover gives in his *Memoirs*, there is considerable evidence that between 1907 and 1914 he faced a dilemma: a conflict between his desires and sense of duty, on the one hand, and his diffidence, shyness, and acute sense of privacy, on the other. As an engineer, he was wearying of money-making and desirous of fulfilling the obligation to "larger service" that was strongly rooted in the ethic of his rapidly expanding profession.[27] As an aspiring "universal man," an autodidact widely read in the literature, history, and philosophy of many nations, an amateur archaeologist of considerable skill, and a capable scholar of mining history and practice, he also viewed government and politics as a new outlet for his amazing energy and a new challenge to his abilities.[28] And finally, as a man who had earned his fortune abroad and moved chiefly in Stanford, mining, and London social circles, he hungered for wider recognition within the United States. As he wrote to a friend at the time:

> The American is always an alien abroad. He can never assimilate. Nor do other peoples ever accept him otherwise than as a foreigner. His heart is in his own country. Yet there is less and less of a niche for him when he returns.
> One feels that one should have built one's fortune in America. It might have been less imposing. Yet one would be among one's own people; and the esteem that one hopes to build among one's associates would not be wasted by leaving it and them behind, only to go home later and then try to build it again.[29]

All of these considerations pulled him toward entry into public life. Yet he found it very difficult to make that entry, chiefly because his social inhibitions and lack of political skills kept him from publicizing himself and becoming "available" in the usual manner, through public appearances and speech-making. In an unpublished memoir, Victoria Allen, wife of Associated Press correspondent Ben S. Allen, recalls that Hoover was so frightened at the prospect of delivering his first public address before the American Navy League in London that he almost neglected to come to the affair. Her husband, a Stanford man who had become well acquainted with Hoover in London, was finally sent to fetch him in time for his speech; and once on the platform, he spoke in "halting sentences" with "every expression indicating diffidence and embarrassment." In content, as her husband remembered it, "the speech was good; in form it was terrible." Nor could anyone ever convince him "that his future Chief did not remember to forget his first speaking engagement."[30]

The Allen memoir also reveals how Hoover contemplated resolving this dilemma, how he hoped to become influential in the United States without subjecting himself to public exposure. The solution, as he evidently saw it in 1914, was a "behind the scenes" approach through the direction of newspapers in California. Through newspaper ownership and editorial expression, he could avoid the exposure that was so abhorrent to him, yet at the same time, by influencing public opinion, he could achieve some control over the shaping of policies. In any event, correspondence between Mrs. Allen and her husband, who was with Hoover in London in the spring of 1914, demonstrates that in her words, "vast as his mining ventures were . . . , Mr. Hoover had made plans to return to California to devote his splendid talents to Stanford University and his home state. He clearly envisioned the direction of more than one paper and entrance into public life."[31] Shortly thereafter Hoover was negotiating, through Allen, for the purchase of the Sacramento *Union,* which the latter would manage for him. Though the war disrupted these plans and Allen came to work with Hoover in the Commission for the Relief of Belgium,[32] it seems clear that, some months before the outbreak of international conflict "shaped Hoover's destiny for him," he had decided that his long-sought-after avenue to influence in the United States was through the press.

That Hoover should have arrived at such a decision is not surprising when one appreciates the literary dimension of his professional achievement and success. A large measure of his renown within the mining profession had been established in the pages of the mining press where, from 1896 through 1912, his articles, letters, and interviews on the geological, economic, and administrative aspects of mining appeared frequently and often stimulated wide-ranging discussion.[33] In the publications of Thomas A. Rickard and his cousin Edgar Rickard, editor and publisher respectively of the influential *Engineering and Mining Journal,* the *Mining Magazine,* and the *Mining and Scientific Press,* he had found an especially resonant sounding-board for his views—views that he hoped would help bring efficiency, stability, and honesty to the chaotic and often scandal-ridden industry.[34] Edgar Rickard, who became an intimate acquaintance of Hoover in London and in 1914 would leave technical publishing to become his closest and longest-serving administrative publicist and all-round aide, had assisted him in the publication and distribution of his *Agricola,*[35] which T. A. Rickard celebrated as having established the learned engineer as "the world's greatest authority" on the history of mining.[36]

In early 1914, evidently, Hoover contemplated exerting influence upon national social and economic questions via the popular press as he had upon the mining industry through its technical journals. And for shaping public opinion via the daily press, he was not inexperienced, for, as we shall see in the next chapter, during the preceding two years, he had been directing a remarkably energetic and skillful press campaign from behind the scenes in London, a campaign on behalf of the Panama-Pacific Exposition.

1. In a prefatory comment upon the pre-1914 section of the first volume of his *Memoirs*, Hoover notes: "This portion was not originally intended for publication. Mrs. Hoover and I always believed the incidents of our family life were our sole possession." It was only to counteract the spread of "myths"—"good and bad" —about his early career that he decided to publish this material (Herbert Clark Hoover, *The Memoirs of Herbert Hoover, 1874-1920:Years of Adventure*, 1:v). Nevertheless, this section, with its heavy emphasis on "constructive works," reveals little of the personality of the writer or the formative influences working upon him. As noted above, the papers at the Herbert Hoover Presidential Library pertaining to this period of his life are still restricted.

2. Henry F. Pringle, "Hoover: An Enigma Easily Misunderstood," pp. 133-34. Other anecdotal sketches of Hoover's personality often suggest an intense nervous energy manifested by his jingling of coins in his pants pockets or rapid pacing back and forth before the visitor, acquaintance, interviewer, and so on.

3. David Hinshaw, *Herbert Hoover: American Quaker*, pp. 26-27.

4. Eugene Lyons, *Our Unknown Ex-President: A Portrait of Herbert Hoover*, p. 71.

5. Will Irwin, *Herbert Hoover: A Reminiscent Biography*, p. 43; William Hard, *Who's Hoover?*, pp. 22-23.

6. Louis Thomas Jones, *The Quakers of Iowa*, pp. 258-81.

7. Hoover's mother was an active Quakeress in prohibition campaigns and a frequent speaker in meetings. Strict in her observation of the Quaker Query prohibiting "pernicious books and corrupt conversation" in the home, she forbade her children to read even the genteel children's magazine *Youth's Companion*. Hoover also refers to his resistance to the repressive atmosphere of chores and "abundant religious occasions" that existed in the home of his uncle in Oregon with whom he lived from age 10 to 17 (Hoover, *Memoirs*, 1:1-11). Although Hoover was aware, and even lightheartedly critical at times, of the oppressiveness of his religious upbringing, it nonetheless left an imprint upon his personality.

8. Jones, *The Quakers of Iowa*, pp. 289-290; Hinshaw, *Herbert Hoover: American Quaker*, p. 45.

9. Irwin, *Herbert Hoover*, pp. 8, 21.

10. 1:10.

11. William Hard, *Who's Hoover?*, pp. 19-20.

12. Hoover, *Memoirs*, 1:14.

13. Ibid., pp. 23-24. In time, in the years before he entered public life, Hoover

overcame this writing problem. The prose of his correspondence and public statements, very little of it "ghost-written," became forceful and lucid, though occasionally marred by awkward construction and phrasing.

14. Ibid., p. 22.

15. Ibid.; Irwin, *Herbert Hoover*, pp. 54-55; Hard, *Who's Hoover?*, pp. 54-58; Ray Lyman Wilbur, *The Memoirs of Ray Lyman Wilbur*, p. 63; David Starr Jordan, "Interesting Westerners," p. 1776.

16. Irwin, a class behind Hoover at Stanford, recalled that "'popularity' [was] not exactly the word for his reaction and influence on his fellows. A better word, probably, would [have been] 'standing.' . . . 'Here I was,' [he quotes Hinsdale as saying] 'older . . . and better at expressing myself. But whenever I came to Hoover, with a suggestion or a proposal, I found myself wondering what he'd think —as though he were my major professor'" (Irwin, *Herbert Hoover*, p. 54). Irwin in his autobiography states that though he knew Hoover possessed an "extraordinary mind," he "would have laughed" if anyone had suggested he might become president of the United States. Presidential material consisted of men "like Hugh Brown or John M. Switzer, who were going in for law and exhorted powerfully on the debating teams!" (Irwin, *The Making of a Reporter*, p. 17).

17. Alexander L. George, "Power As a Compensatory Value for Political Leaders," p. 45.

18. The exact amount of Hoover's fortune at its peak in 1914 has long been a subject of controversy. Late in his presidency when accusations of financial turpitude were being hurled at Hoover from a number of quarters, *Fortune* magazine presented what it called the "ascertainable facts" on the matter. Presenting a chart purporting to account for Hoover's earnings from a score of mines around the world, *Fortune* calculated that, in 1914, the engineer-promoter's wealth stood in excess of four million dollars ("The President's Fortune," *Fortune*, [August, 1932], p. 32). However, in the handwritten, autobiographical statement referred to above, Hoover estimates his fortune in 1914 to have been around thirty million dollars. The war, he says, "crushed this fortune down by 95% . . . [leaving] under one million dollars [but enough] not only to live upon but to further diminish by the necessities of charity" (undated, autobiographical statement, Box 1-Q/279, HHP, HHPL).

19. Geoffrey Blainey, *The Rush That Never Ended: A History of Australian Mining*, pp. 202, 265-66, 277.

20. Hoover, *Memoirs*, 1:128-30.

21. Vernon Kellogg, *Herbert Hoover: The Man and His Work*, p. 137; Hard, *Who's Hoover?*, pp. 115-17; Hinshaw, *Herbert Hoover: American Quaker*, pp. 67-72.

22. Hoover, *The Memoirs of Herbert Hoover, 1920-1933: The Cabinet and the Presidency*, 2:v-vi.

23. David Starr Jordan, *The Days of a Man*, 2:223.

24. Henry F. Pringle, *The Life and Times of William H. Taft*, 2:613-14.

25. Quoted in Irwin, *Herbert Hoover*, p. 123; *The Making of a Reporter*, pp. 182-83.

26. Mary Austin, *Earth Horizon*, p. 322; Austin, "Hoover and Johnson: West Is West," p. 643.

27. It has been commonly asserted that Quaker humanitarianism was the "dominant influence which started Hoover on his public career" in 1914 (cf. Hinshaw, *Herbert Hoover*, pp. 71-76). I have found nothing in Hoover's published writings or papers to substantiate this view and feel a much better case can be made

for the influence upon him of the ethic of the engineer. The professional journals of engineering societies in the late nineteenth and early twentieth centuries frequently referred to the engineer's reward for his services as a " 'competence' an adequate means for living comfortably, but without excess." As the first president of the American Society of Mechanical Engineers wrote in 1881, the engineer's task was not "the piling of gold and silver in treasury vaults, and not the aggregation of fictitious values on Wall Street," but the production of "durable materials," essential to the well-being of society (quoted in Samuel Haber, *Efficiency and Uplift: Scientific Management in the Progressive Era, 1890-1920*, pp. 10-11). Hoover, as a member of the American Society of Civil Engineers, the Engineers Club of San Francisco, and the American Institute of Mining Engineers (which offered him its presidency in 1914), fully subscribed to this ethic and its political overtones. In the first volume of his *Memoirs*, written in the period 1915-16, he wrote: "To the engineer falls the job of clothing the bare bones of science with life, comfort and hope. . . . With the industrial revolution and the advancement of engineers to the administration of industry as well as its technical direction, the governmental, economic and social impacts upon the engineers have steadily increased. Once, lawyers were the only professional men whose contacts with the problems of government led them on to positions of public responsibility. From the point of view of accuracy and intellectual honesty the more men of engineering background who become public officials, the better for representative government" (p. 133).

28. Hoover once expressed his regret to Irwin that he had had to earn his living while going to college. He was sure he would have made himself "a better all-round man if [he] hadn't lost so much time just making a living" (quoted in Irwin, *Herbert Hoover*, p. 68). Aware that his failure at Stanford to achieve much in the way of a liberal education, he undertook, in the years 1904 to 1907, a "reeducation of myself—history, economics, sociology, politics, [and] government. [I] read literally several thousand books giving at least two hours nightly and all spare time on long voyages" (undated, autobiographical statement, Box 1-Q/279, HHP, HHPL). In his *Memoirs*, he specifies some of the figures he read at this time: Balzac, Dumas, Zola, Victor Hugo, Rousseau, Montaigne, Voltaire, Mirabeau, the Encyclopedists, Confucius, Mencius, Plato, Shakespeare, Schiller, Goethe (1:40, 47). In the years 1907-12, he also participated in archeological digs in Egypt and northern Italy that shed new light upon the history of the ancient Egyptian and Roman empires. With the assistance of his wife, he made the first translation from Latin to English of Agricola's *De Re Metallica*, a sixteenth-century compilation of Renaissance knowledge of mining and industrial chemistry. The introduction to this work and the numerous explanatory footnotes designed to place Agricola's work in its proper historical perspective display much scholarly erudition. A series of lectures on mining engineering that Hoover delivered at Columbia and Stanford in 1909 were published in the same year as *Principles of Mining*—a work that remained a standard text in the field for many years (ibid., 1:97-98, 117-19).

29. Quoted in Hard, *Who's Hoover?*, pp. 65-66.

30. Victoria Allen, "The Outside Man," (unpublished, undated), 1:74-75, Ben Allen Papers, Herbert Hoover Presidential Library. Not until long after his presidential years was Hoover able to overcome his inhibitions well enough to deliver an effective speech. A common observation of friendly commentators upon the quality of his leadership was that for all his mastery over men in small groups, Hoover was simply incapacitated by large audiences. Theodore Joslin, his presidential press secretary, has written that though Hoover could "invariably influence" and "win over" opponents seated in front of him in conference, "he did not appear to such advantage before a large audience. His arguments were as sound, but he did

not quite get them over. He was not quite his true self in public. Perhaps it was because he always read from manuscript and talked in a monotone that was tiring, instead of with the emphasis that marked his private, informal conversations" (Theodore Joslin, *Hoover off the Record*, p. 7). Henry Pringle, who heard Hoover speak frequently in the 1920s, called him one of the most "lamentably bad public speakers in the United States" and probably the most deficient in the art ever to aspire to the Presidency. Pringle noted that before small groups he did well, but before large audiences "inhibitions seem to rise in his throat and to choke his vocal chords. One hand is kept in his pocket, usually jingling [coins] placed there to ease his nerves. He has not a single gesture. . . . He reads—his chin down against his shirt front—rapidly and quite without expression" ("Hoover: An Enigma Easily Misunderstood," p. 131). On this same point, see also: Hans V. Kaltenborn, *Fifty Fabulous Years, 1900-1950: A Personal Review by H. V. Kaltenborn* (New York, 1950), p. 159; Irwin, "Herbert Hoover: An Intimate Portrait," p. 126; William Allen White, *The Autobiography of William Allen White*, p. 515; Dr. Edgar Robinson, Professor Emeritus, Stanford University, interviewed by Raymond Henle, Director, Herbert Hoover Oral History Program, September 13, 1967, p. 4, HHPL.

31.   Allen, "The Outside Man," 1:105. Mary Austin also recalls that Hoover expressed to her an interest in buying a newspaper as a way of "getting into something" in the United States (*Earth Horizon*, p. 322).

32.   Hoover did buy the *Union* in 1919, and Allen became his managing editor. In the same year, he purchased an interest in the Washington *Herald*. He liquidated both interests in 1921 ("Hearst Buys *Herald* in Washington," p. 16; "Sacramento *Union* is Sold by Allen," p. 37). Knowledge of his purchasing of these papers seems to have given rise initially to the notion that Hoover was ambitious for the presidency and trying to use publicity to achieve it. See, for instance, Josephus Daniels, *The Wilson Era: Years of War and After, 1917-1923*, p. 319, and Donald Wilhelm, "If He Were President," p. 210.

33.   In March, 1914, Hoover became the first recipient of the Mining and Metallurgical Society's gold metal award presented annually to an eminent mining engineer. Hoover's award was for "distinguished contributions to the literature of mining" ("The Hoover Dinner," *Engineering and Mining Journal* 97 [March 14, 1914]: 577). The findings of a student of Hoover's early career indicate that his views were published in as many as twenty different technical journals—journals located in England, the United States, Australia, and China (David Burner, "Primary Sources on Herbert Hoover's Business Career," Paper Read at the Southwest Social Science Association, March, 1970, Dallas, Texas).

34.   "The Hoover Dinner," p. 577; T. A. Rickard, *Interviews with Mining Engineers* (San Francisco, 1922), pp. 534, 541; Hoover, "Some Notes on Crossings," *Mining and Scientific Press* 72 (February 29, 1896): 166; "The Geology of the Four-Mile Placer Mining District, Colorado," *Engineering and Mining Journal* 63 (May 22, 1897): 510; "Mining and Melting Gold Ores in Western Australia," *EMJ* 66 (December 17, 1898): 725; "Present Situation of the Mining Industry in China," *EMJ* 69 (May 26, 1900): 619-20; "The Kaiping Coal Mines and Coal Field, Chible Province, North China," *EMJ* 74 (August 2, 1902): 149; "Gold Mining in Western Australia in 1902," *EMJ* 75 (January 3, 1903): 18; "The Treatment of Sulfo-Telluride Ores at Kalgoorlie," *EMJ* 76 (August 1, 1903): 156; "Permanence in Depth in Kalgoorlie," *EMJ* 76 (October 31, 1903): 655; "The Economic Ratio of Treatment Capacity to Ore Reserves," *EMJ* 76 (March 24, 1904): 475; "The Valuation of Gold Mines," *EMJ* 76 (May 19, 1904): 801; "West Australian Gold Mining in 1905," *EMJ* 76 (January 20, 1906): 136; "Counsels of Imperfection," *Mining Magazine* 2 (January, 1910): 40-41; "Economics of a Boom," *MM* 6 (May, 1912); "Australian Min-

ing Laws," *MSP* 104 (May 25, 1912): 731; "Mine Valuation and Mine Finance," *MM* 7 (October, 1912).

35. Hoover, *Memoirs*, 1:118, 122-23; "Rickard, Edgar," *Belgian and American C.R.B. Fellows 1920-1950: Biographical Dictionary* (New York, 1950), p. 179.

36. EMJ 95 (February 22, 1913): 436.

2 Selling the Panama-Pacific Exposition

AN AUTHOR HIMSELF, occasional contributor to the nontechnical press,[1] and avid reader of current affairs, Herbert Hoover had become well acquainted with the daily and periodical literature of the United States, Australia, and England. As early as 1898 as a mine manager in Western Australia, he had begun subscribing to a score of "papers and magazines" among them the *Century, Strand, Windsor, Harper's Magazine, Pearson's Monthly Magazine, Review of Reviews, Australian, Punch, Illustrated London News, Graphic, Scientific American,* and *Pall Mall Magazine.*[2] In addition, he had frequently enjoyed the company of American and English writers and newspapermen at Red House, his London home. He had associated with them during the long hours at sea between mining ventures,[3] and with some of them he had developed close ties. Mary Austin and Will Irwin, for example, had become established members of the Hoover circle; and with Robert M. Collins, head of the London office of the Associated Press and the man to whom he owed his valuable connection with Ben Allen, he had a long friendship dating back to 1900, when he had sheltered Collins and other American correspondents in his residence at Tientsin during the Boxer Rebellion.[4] From such extensive reading and personal contacts, he had learned a good deal about the press and its influence.

That by 1912 he believed himself capable of putting this knowledge to use is also evident from extensive correspondence between himself and the San Francisco promoters of the Panama-Pacific

Exposition. This correspondence, covering the period from July, 1912, through August, 1914, demonstrates Hoover's deep belief in the power of public opinion and the manner in which he felt it could be mobilized to effect certain desired results. It is also significant in that it reveals Hoover's characteristic behind-the-scenes style of action, his inclination always to work through influential public men and journalists while keeping himself in the background. In it, one can study the first major "public" activity of his career, which, in turn, constitutes a kind of "case study" of the public relations style that typified his later administrative work. And for this reason, his work on behalf of the Exposition, will be examined in some detail.

In April, 1912, Hoover had volunteered his services to the organizers of the Exposition, scheduled to run in San Francisco from February through December, 1915. The idea for this was an old one, dating back to 1904; but not until 1910, when the Exposition's Committee on Permanent Organization established a corporation called the Panama-Pacific International Exposition, had any concrete plans developed. The intention, once these had taken shape, was to commemorate the 400th anniversary of Balboa's discovery of the Pacific Ocean, celebrate the opening of the Panama Canal, and, of central concern to the Exposition's promoters, draw international commercial attention to the Pacific Coast and to the Bay Area specifically. Federal support had also been quickly secured. In December, 1911, after the organizers of the Exposition had demonstrated that they could raise the $15 million deemed necessary to host the event, Congress had passed a joint resolution authorizing President Taft to invite foreign countries to participate. This Taft had done in February, 1912, and two months later, a "Commission Extraordinary to Europe," formed by the Exposition's organizers and armed with credentials making it the official representative of the United States, had embarked for Europe to drum up support for the fair in European capitals. In London, the responsibility for doing this had fallen upon Dr. Frederick J. V. Skiff, and it was Skiff who was approached by "a quiet, pleasant-mannered young man [who] evinced a desire to help in the promotion of so constructive and beneficial an enterprise." At the time, he recalled, he had "never heard of Herbert Clark Hoover, but he seemed eager to help."[5] Thus it was that Hoover, "a Californian in London" as he called himself,[6] became an overseas agent of the Panama-Pacific Exposition and found his first opportunity to be of service to his state and nation.

Once involved, it was not long before he was designing schemes to promote the Exposition in England and attempting to carry them out. Aware that influential political and social leaders in London life regarded the Exposition "as apparently a case of a commercial Exposition of the usual order . . . and therefore not to be taken seriously," he sounded out the San Francisco-based president of the Exposition, Charles C. Moore, on the possibility of overcoming this attitude by inviting King George V to attend the fair and having him travel to San Francisco by way of the Panama Canal. If this could be done, he reasoned, it would bring the Exposition a tremendous amount of publicity and give to it an authentic international flavor. But in order to realize it, he knew, "the groundwork would have to be prepared behind the throne," for without such preparation, "an open and overt proposal of this kind would undoubtedly meet with refusal." He therefore suggested that the "matter be handled with discretion through private English hands," whom he knew to be sympathetic.[7] And once Moore had encouraged him by telegram to pursue the plan, he undertook private discussions with Arthur Balfour, the former Conservative prime minister, discussions in which he argued, in particular, that a royal visit to the Exposition would "cement and increase" the growing good feeling between the United States and Britain, "advance the education of our people" in international affairs, and perhaps move Americans away from their "sacred policy of political isolation," especially if it could demonstrate to them that, in a world of shrinking markets and increasing international instability, "the only certain and enduring alliance would be between peoples of the same race."[8] Impressed with Hoover's arguments, Balfour agreed to work, in his own words, "to develop sentiment amongst important people." At the same time, feeling himself a "missionary in the matter . . . stimulating [others] to action," Hoover also arranged for some of his English friends to bring the project to the attention of Sir Edward Grey, the foreign minister in the incumbent Liberal government, who, once familiarized with it, was reported to be "warmly in favour of such a proposal, in his personal capacity, as distinguished from his official position."[9] And finally, having set in motion such pressures from "behind the throne," Hoover turned for further aid to the American Committee for the Celebration of the Hundred Years of Peace Among the English Speaking Peoples. In the autumn of 1912, this group adopted the "illustrious visitor" project and joined forces with Hoover in trying to realize it.[10]

Meanwhile, in conjunction with his visitation project, Hoover had set out to bring the right type of newspaper publicity to the Exposition. And again, one should note, he employed a behind-the-scenes approach, one that worked through Robert P. Porter, a veteran American correspondent and world traveler, who in 1912 was an associate editor of the London *Times* in charge of the Special Supplement Department,[11] and who had also become a good friend of Hoover during the latter's London years, the first, in fact, of a long line of journalists with whom Hoover would become well acquainted and upon whom he would come to rely in the course of his varied administrative career. In July, 1912, Hoover prevailed upon Porter to publish an interview with an Exposition official whose business, he thought, was "of some public interest in this country," would "form good news material," and, from Hoover's own point of view, would provide a "news feature" that he could exploit to publicize the "international character" of the Exposition.[12] At the same time, he interested Porter in the idea of preparing and publishing a special supplement in the *Times*, a project that won Moore's enthusiastic approval, so much so that Porter, in September, 1912, made plans to travel to California to gather materials and Hoover offered further advice on what the special number should stress. Its theme, as he saw it, should not be "land boosting," but rather "the Panama Canal and the Exposition itself"; and it should be a "literary effort along historical, romantic, and economic lines"—"a higher type of production" than the usual booster sheets.[13]

In the fall and winter of 1912-13, however, the plans that Hoover had laid so well began to go awry. Through no fault of his own, both the "illustrious visitor" and the "special supplement" projects began to lose the support that he had cultivated so assiduously during the previous summer. The trouble stemmed from the fact that in August, 1912, Congress, in violation of the spirit of the 1901 Hay-Pauncefote Treaty, had exempted American ships using the Panama Canal from toll payment; and despite British protests that such legislation violated the "equality" clause of the treaty, neither President Taft nor presidential candidates Woodrow Wilson and Theodore Roosevelt would criticize it.[14] As knowledge of the American action spread in England, British public sentiment became inflamed; and to some extent, refusal to participate in the San Francisco Exposition, which, it should be remembered, had been conceived in part as a celebration of the opening of the canal, became a means by which the British could retaliate against the discriminatory tolls legislation. In any event, by late October, 1912, Hoover had learned that the editorial staff of the *Times* was now divided over "the desirability of bringing out a Panama Canal number in face of the recent legislation."[15]

Confronted with this setback, Hoover tried his best to counteract it. He wrote to Porter arguing that the legislation was "not anti-English in its character." It was merely "a part of the regular propaganda which necessarily prevails prior to Presidential election," a part, as he put it, of the ancient American political strategy of "twisting the lion's tail." For this reason, he urged that the *Times* "duly proceed with the job" of the special supplement, and in doing so, might use it to discuss the whole matter "so long as it was done in a judicial and not in an anti-American manner."[16] Such arguments, though, went unheeded. As he wrote to Moore in February, 1913, he had had "two or three interviews with the *Times* staff about the special edition, but the Panama position hangs as a sort of cloud over everything here and I have as yet been unable to get anything finally forward."[17] Nor was he able to advance the "illustrious visitor" scheme. On this, he could "only repeat" that "it all comes back to the same old stone wall . . . that is that al-

though personal sentiment is greatly in favour of such a move, absolutely nothing can be done in an overt manner until the Canal
Dues question is shelved in some way or other."[18]

With his "indirect approach" immobilized by the Panama question, Hoover now contemplated a publicity campaign to attack the
problem directly. Feeling that the withholding of formal British
recognition of the Exposition because of the tolls issue was "extremely small politics" and something "the British public in general would not stand for," he pondered getting "the subject raised
in the press by questions in Parliament and resolutions in the
Chambers of Commerce through friends." Moore, though, was
fearful that such actions, by appearing to be intervening in British
political life, would further jeopardize Exposition interests; and
in view of such fears, Hoover did not proceed. "I do not know
that such a policy is at all wise," he wrote, "and I would not do
anything on these lines without some hint from your end," at least
nothing beyond what could be initiated "simply as a private individual among my own friends."[19]

In June, 1913, Hoover finally did succeed in getting the *Times*
editorial staff to issue the special number, an event, he hoped, that
"would come nearer breaking through the newspaper boycott than
anything else which [could] possibly be devised."[20] Its effects, however, were disappointing and were soon offset by another setback.
On August 6, Foreign Minister Grey officially announced in the
House of Commons that the British government would not accept
President Taft's invitation. The principal reasons given for the refusal were that the estimated government expenditure would be
out of proportion to any commercial gain resulting from participation and that inquiries in commercial centers in the United Kingdom did not indicate any desire for participation.[21]

With the British government's position now clearly stated, Hoover again recommended to Moore, more forcefully than previously, a widespread press campaign to induce the government to
change its mind. On August 10, he wired Moore:

My view is failure to secure British participation largely due entire lack of publicity and outside pushing at this. . . . If expo-

sition could see way to expend moderate amount on publicity here putting forward relations Pacific Coast market to British manufacturers after opening of Canal would have ultimate effect. If Porter is with you suggest you discuss frankly with him securing publicity campaign he is most loyal American and has better knowledge of Press position here than any one in England.[22]

At the same time, bolstered with trade statistics supplied by the American ambassador to England, Walter Hines Page, Hoover wrote to the *Times*, arguing that the Panama Canal had opened a vast new trading market on the North American Pacific Coast that the British manufacturer could profitably penetrate. The Panama-Pacific Exposition, he continued, would greatly benefit the manufacturer by giving him an opportunity to acquaint Americans with his wares, and apparently, the *Times* agreed. On August 20, it came out with a strong editorial favoring British acceptance. On the same date, Hoover wired Moore asking what arrangements he had made "regarding the press campaign" and noting that it was important to "keep in motion [the] discussion now going on."[23] Then having received no response, he embarked upon a new tack, one that would advance the cause of the Exposition and continue the agitation through organizing a purely British committee, composed of prominent members of Parliament and industrialists. This he suggested to Moore, and when the latter failed to show interest, Hoover's patience temporarily gave way. On September 4, he wrote testily to a sympathetic official of the Exposition, John Barneson: "I am simply having to say [to English contacts] that I am not authorized to do anything. The whole position is disheartening when one can see with the utmost clearness where things are going to. . . . I simply intend to let matters take their course. I cannot, with any sense of personal dignity, further impose my views on the Exposition, nor am I looking for more jobs in this world nor honours of this kind."[24]

This fit of pique, however, quickly abated. Several days later Hoover was back at work organizing the "British Committee" that would carry on the fight for formal government participation in the Exposition. With the approval of several Exposition representatives currently in London, among them Skiff and Barneson, and with the cooperation of a few British M.P.'s and industrialists who desired participation, he began by engaging William A. M. Goode as secretary of the British Committee for the Panama-Pacific Exposition. Goode, like Porter, was a veteran journalist and editor with extensive newspaper experience in both the United States and England.[25] As news editor of the London *Standard* from 1904 to 1910 and joint news editor of the *Daily Mail* since 1911, he was ideally equipped, in Hoover's mind, to direct pro-Exposition publicity in the English press. Through Goode, Hoover also hoped to enlarge the original committee, chiefly by distributing propaganda circulars to leading politicians and businessmen who might be persuaded to challenge the government's decision on economic grounds. For these purposes, an office was soon opened, with Hoover providing the necessary money, apparently out of his own pocket.[26] And shortly thereafter, Moore came around. Learning of Skiff's approval and faced with a *fait accompli* in any case, he gave his telegraphic assent to the committee and authorized an expenditure for it of $4,500 out of Exposition funds.[27] Apparently, he now agreed with Hoover, who, on September 19, had summed up the reasons for, and advantages of working through, a British Committee. "After innumerable interviews with Barneson, Skiff . . . and various others of your birds of flight on this side," he wrote, "they all seem to come to the conclusion that my recommendation as to the present situation is the only one to adhere to." And this, "in simplified form," was:

1.   That a purely British movement should be stimulated to form initially a Provisional Committee of most eminent men, and later a General Committee embracing every branch of influence, the sole object of which Committee is to secure Government participation.

2.   That the Panama Pacific, in all of its manifestations by way of agents, should get down out of Great Britain at the earliest possible moment, in order that there be no charge of intrigue on the part of the Exposition itself, and so that the Englishmen who are taking the matter up can go at it conscientiously as their own movement, initiated and controlled by themselves.[28]

Hoover's desire to get all "outside" Exposition agents out of Great Britain, himself excepted, was prompted by the maladroit promotional work of one J. B. Lester, an Exposition commissioner, whose efforts on behalf of the Exposition in London in early September Hoover resented because they rivaled his own and because they were so inept. Against Hoover's judgment, Lester had arranged that the government's Board of Trade make another survey of commercial opinion in England—his feeling being that, on this occasion, it would reveal overwhelming sentiment for participation. Hoover had argued futilely that this "might be absolutely fatal . . . because if the inquiry [again] came out unfavourably we could make Committees and raise agitation until we were blind because the Government, having been further substantiated in their view as to the wishes of the commercial community, [would] never move hand or foot."[29] When Hoover's fears materialized and the new survey again indicated little commercial interest, he wrote to Skiff that it was "distinctly dangerous to have this gentleman remain in England."[30] He also complained to Moore about Lester's clumsiness, especially his failure to "cultivate" the manufacturers, who "did not know the real situation." Such a man, he felt, should have been instructed "to do nothing without my approval."[31] And his views did prevail. On October 3, Skiff wrote to Hoover, agreeing with him about Lester and assuring him that the latter was leaving England for the United States.[32]

Having disposed of Lester, Hoover and Goode, working closely but furtively together, proceeded to expand the British committee. During October and early November, they succeeded in placing fifty of England's leading commercial figures on the committee— among them the lord mayor of London, the chairman of the London Chamber of Commerce, the president of the Associated [British] Chambers of Commerce, and the chairmen of the largest manufacturing, steel, and coal companies in the country. Hoover, in a letter to Moore on September 30, reckoned that it was best to begin with the "absolute commercial leaders . . . of largely Liberal complection for it would be easy to get the opponents of the Government and the noodle-headed Peer later." He added with "amusement" that "several Peers had already approached our people and volunteered" but that they were being "kept out of the way" until "the men of stability, who so strongly resent being associated with purely social nobodies, [could] be secured."[33] In the middle of November, the British committee forwarded a memorandum, prepared by Hoover and Goode, to the government, pointing out that participation would cost a good deal less than what the government had originally estimated; that British exports to the Pacific Coast, far greater than the total estimated when the refusal was announced, warranted official participation; and that, since the invitation had been refused, conditions in both the United States and in England had changed considerably as demonstrated by the unexpectedly favorable American tariff legislation and by the rapidly increasing British commercial desire for participation. The memorandum concluded with the request that the government receive a small deputation representing the committee in order that the arguments presented might receive a personal hearing.[34]

While organizing the British committee and preparing the memorandum to the government, Hoover and Goode also "made [their] plunge into publicity," as Hoover referred to their efforts.[35] In October, Goode had enlisted the support of Harold Spender, who, in his view, was "perhaps the strongest" of all writers on "Liberal topics,"[36] and whose varied career, dating back to the 1880s and including personal friendships with Liberal politicians and successive associations with the *Pall Mall Gazette*, *Westminster Gazette*, *Daily Chronicle*, *Manchester Guardian*, and *Daily News*, made him an extremely valuable acquisition.[37] With his assistance, and with the cooperation of Robert Donald, editor of the *Daily Chronicle*, Goode was successful in eliciting favorable editorial comment for the Exposition from newspapers throughout Great Britain.[38]

Through Spender, moreover, and specifically through his connections with Chancellor of the Exchequer David Lloyd-George, Hoover and Goode learned that, just as they had suspected, the real reason for the government's decision was the Panama tolls legislation.[39] Nor, as they subsequently discovered from the same "inside" sources, was this the whole story. A year before, on the initiative of Foreign Minister Grey, England and Germany had made an informal, secret agreement to boycott the Exposition in order to retaliate against the American Panama policy, and the German government now felt honor-bound not to reopen the question until approached by the British.[40] Once in possession of such knowledge, however, Goode was reluctant to use it and favored instead a continuation of the publicity designed to point up the mistaken reasoning behind the government's official position, i.e., that it was not economically feasible to participate in the fair. He feared making the real reason for nonparticipation public knowledge, for as he wrote to Hoover, "I need not dilate upon the effect of the publication [of the existence of the agreement] in America without any simultaneous announcement as to British participation." News of the agreement, "published in distorted version possibly," would take "bitter prominence both here and in the United States."[41]

For several days, Hoover seemed to agree. As he wrote Moore on November 25 and 27, he too favored the continued application of "indirect pressures"; and along this line, he saw to it that a letter warning of the possible consequences of American knowledge of the agreement reached Sir Edward Grey by way of Harold Spender—"a rather dangerous *ballon d'essai*," he admitted to Moore, "but something [had to] be done to force an issue."[42] He also secured Lord Northcliffe's cooperation in "sounding the note [in his newspapers] of German intention to be largely represented, all of which [would be] helpful by way of indirect pressure."[43] Before long, however, he had become impatient with such tactics, and he now decided to open up public discussion of the Panama issue, something he had wanted to do the previous March, and to make the Anglo-German agreement public knowledge. Without receiving Moore's approval, or even informing him of his intent, he broke the story to the press. A letter to his confidant, Barneson, dated December 5, describes his actions and gives a sense of the personal satisfaction he derived from wielding influence from behind the scenes. Indeed, since it reveals much about Hoover's tactical use of public relations, it seems advisable to let him speak for himself:

As to the British participation question generally I have had scarcely a minute to do anything else during the whole of the last month. Goode proved himself, as I anticipated when I recommended his engagement, a very skillful, knowing chap, but lacking in moral courage and requiring a pretty strong guiding hand. My view of general tactics widely differs from his, but I have insisted on having my own way, although I have had to go outside of the Committee business entirely in order to get it.

The point is that we requested the Prime Minister to receive a deputation. Goode dilly-dallied along about this question much longer than was necessary, but having sent the request in, it was my belief that every single gun that we had should be brought to bear, and all at once, because the matter then comes before the whole Cabinet in a form upon which they have got to take some action, considering the importance of our Committee, and from the very minute that this request was sent in we had to turn loose every battery. One of our strongest guns, to my mind, consisted in the gentle exposure of this Anglo-German agreement directed against the San Francisco Exposition and other American matters. Goode, Lipton [an original Committee member and organizer], and others were in a funk about having anything of this kind published, and I have taken it upon myself to indirectly expose the whole blooming situation.

I have done this in three ways: First, I got my friend here who is head of the Associated Press in Europe to have their people in Berlin corroborate the existence of such an agreement through Ballin [an Exposition agent working in Germany], and then send [a] dispatch to London through Reuters. Second, I go to the Editor of the "Times," through my old friend Porter, and put the situation to him, and the necessity for his handling it with diplomatic care; and Third, I get Page to let the fact leak out from the State Department in Washington. All this has created a mild sensation, and whereas a good many people are somewhat aggravated to think that the matter has become public, I have not the slightest doubt in my own mind that it will have a great effect. . . .

The fact is, my old friend, that while I have a great appreciation of these smooth, diplomatic folk who accomplish things by innocent and mild manners, there are times in the history of every transaction when a little sprinkling of fighting blood like you possess is more good than a thousand carefully drawn up letters.[44]

On the same day that he was writing Barneson the above letter, Hoover wired Moore that he was sailing for New York the next day, "having brought every pressure and device to bear that we can imagine."[45] In addition to those described, he had made one last effort, a suggestion to Ambassador Page that he ask the French government "to intervene to break down the silly diplomatic impasse at which we have arrived."[46] All of these strategems, however, failed. On December 19, Goode wired Hoover in New York that he had just received word from Prime Minister Henry Asquith's personal secretary, Bonham Carter, that the cabinet, upon consideration of the committee's memorandum, were unable to modify their previous decision and felt that "no good object would be served by receiving a deputation."[47] As the next step, he recommended forming a purely Parliamentary committee to carry on the fight, as there seemed to be some sentiment for this in the House of Commons. Hoover wired his approval, and while this new approach was taking shape, he kept himself busy in the United States, chiefly in instigating publicity designed to counteract the demoralizing news of England's and Germany's joint refusal to participate.

In early January, 1914, Goode sent Hoover several press clippings from English newspapers, charging that Hoover had been responsible for "leaking" the news of the Anglo-German agreement. Hoover replied without acknowledging his actions. He stated simply that Lord Grey had been warned about anti-English feeling arising in the United States should the agreement become known there, and now that such hostility had developed, he was trying to allay it through a press campaign, designed to show that the Anglo-German agreement was concerned with other matters and was not really anti-Exposition in character. He felt, moreover, that he was succeeding, that "the very large publicity I have instigated—and to some extent carried on—on this side" had consolidated "American feeling on behalf of the Exposition."[48] A week later, while complaining to Ben Allen that the London *Times* was unfairly trying to "lay the story [of the agreement] on me exclusively," he noted that "the publicity that was got out of this affair on this side has quite put the Exposition on its feet so far as American sentiment is concerned and if I have to be offered up as a sacrifice on this altar I can stand it."[49] For a man who delighted in "bold" action and seemed to take pride in his possession of "moral courage," Hoover thus proved strikingly reluctant to accept responsibility—even to his closest friends and associates—for the public furor created by his display of "fighting blood." His behavior in this instance—"bold action" followed by extreme sensitivity to public exposure—is very revealing of his assertive yet, at the same time, retiring personality.

Though all of Hoover's efforts on behalf of the Panama-Pacific Exposition in Great Britain failed to achieve their ultimate objective, it has seemed to me important to pay close attention to this episode in his life, occurring, as it did, at the watershed between his private and public careers. For although the British Liberal government never did recognize the Exposition, Hoover was convinced that his public relations schemes had proven successful. Had it not been for such extraordinary events as near domestic civil strife in England in the spring of 1914, followed by the outbreak of World War I in the summer of that year, his tactics probably would have attained their end. In April, 1914, Goode, his industrious publicist in London, had succeeded in getting a majority of the members of the House of Commons to petition the government to change its position on the Exposition question. And though the harried government still would not change its position, Hoover could point with pride to the massive shift in influential English opinion that his publicity work had effected in the two preceding years.[50]

In addition to stimulating Hoover's growing confidence in the efficacy of publicity techniques, the Panama-Pacific episode is also significant for what it reveals of Hoover the man. For the individual involved here was a much more complex figure than that suggested by the "legend" of the unwitting, altruistic businessman who "accidentally" entered and ascended in public life. In his extensive correspondence, we catch a glimpse of his self-confident assertiveness, his pleasure and excitement in taking part in a large "public" venture, his knowledge of the international political econ-

omy, and his hitherto unsuspected stature among powerful seg-
ments of English society as well as at the American embassy in
London. Here clearly was a man "of large affairs," a man who would
want to be of "larger service" to his native society, yet one who,
for all his assertiveness, even aggressiveness at times, preferred to
operate behind "front men" in the carrying out of his schemes.
Though, in his view, a "behind the scenes" strategy was required
by the circumstances of English politics, it was nevertheless a
strategy especially fitted to the requirements of his personality and
one that would become his routine modus operandi in later years.
Shy, introverted, and always extremely sensitive to criticism, he
used journalists and eminent men to achieve his ends, just as he
would do later in American public life, and by doing so, was able
to maintain his personal privacy and minimize the public exposure that was so discomfiting to him. Given his social inhibitions
against offering personal leadership, it is understandable that
Hoover, for all his desire to enter public life and to move men and
events, would have had difficulty doing so prior to 1914. And given
his successful dealings with newspapermen and editors in London
in the Exposition episode, it is also understandable that early in
1914 he would be contemplating newspaper ownership as a way of
wielding influence in the United States. When the Great War
called Hoover to the new work he had long been seeking, he was
well aware from personal experience of the potential assistance that
the press could provide; and for him, the aggressive introvert, publicity machines and public relations techniques, tactics similar to
those he had used in London in 1913-14, would become indispensable.

1. See for instance, Herbert Hoover, "The Training of the Mining Engineer,"
Science: A Weekly Journal Devoted to the Advancement of Science 20 (November
25, 1904): 716-19, in which he argued for "a thoroughly broad groundwork of education in the humanities, as well as the sciences, prior to . . . entrance to the technical schools"; also, Hoover, "The Future Output of Gold," New York *Sun*, Sept. 8,
1912.

2. "Department of Mines—Herbert Hoover's Letterbook, 1898–March, 1899,"
Microfilm 70/467, Western Australia, Herbert Hoover Presidential Library.

3. Frederick Palmer, *With My Own Eyes: A Personal Story of Battle Years,* pp. 174-75.

4. Herbert Hoover, *The Memoirs of Herbert Hoover, 1874-1920: Years of Adventure,* 1:53; Victoria Allen, "The Outside Man," (unpublished, undated), 1:33, Ben Allen Papers, HHPL.

5. Frank Morton Todd, *The Story of the Exposition,* 1:35, 63, 214-16, and 222-23. Todd's five-volume study does not deal with Hoover's efforts on behalf of the Exposition beyond mentioning the fact of his cooperation. Thus, the Hoover Papers are the sole documentation covering his involvement in the venture.

6. Hoover to Charles C. Moore, June 11, 1912, Pre-Commerce, Panama-Pacific File, HHP, HHPL.

7. Hoover to Moore, July 5, 1912, Pre-Commerce, Panama-Pacific File, HHP, HHPL.

8. Hoover to Moore, July 27, 1912, Pre-Commerce, Panama-Pacific File, HHP, HHPL.

9. Ibid.

10. Hoover to Moore, December 17, 1912, Pre-Commerce, Panama-Pacific File, HHP, HHPL.

11. *Who Was Who, 1916-1928* (London, 1929), p. 349.

12. Hoover to Porter, July 24, 1912, "Panama Pacific International Exposition, Miscellaneous, P-Z," Pre-Commerce, Panama-Pacific File, HHP, HHPL.

13. Hoover to Porter, September 27, 1912, "Panama Pacific International Exposition, Miscellaneous, P-Z," Pre-Commerce, Panama-Pacific File, HHP, HHPL.

14. Alexander De Conde, *A History of American Foreign Policy,* pp. 406-7.

15. Hoover to Porter, October 25, 1912, "Panama Pacific International Exposition, Miscellaneous, P-Z," Pre-Commerce, Panama-Pacific File, HHP, HHPL. In this letter, Hoover correctly predicts that the offensive "section of the act will be ultimately modified by some means." On July 11, 1914, Congress did restore equality of dues payment in the Canal Zone (De Conde, *A History of American Foreign Policy,* p. 407).

16. Hoover to Porter, October 25, 1912, "Panama Pacific International Exposition, Miscellaneous, P-Z," Pre-Commerce, Panama-Pacific File, HHP, HHPL.

17. Hoover to Moore, February 12, 1913, Pre-Commerce, Panama-Pacific File, HHP, HHPL.

18. Hoover to Moore, March 11, 1913, Pre-Commerce, Panama-Pacific File, HHP, HHPL.

19. Ibid.

20. Hoover to Moore, June 19, 1913, Pre-Commerce, Panama-Pacific File, HHP, HHPL.

21. *The Panama-Pacific Exposition: The Facts of the Case* (London, January, 1914), 7, Pre-Commerce, Panama-Pacific File, HHP, HHPL.

22. Hoover to Moore, August 10, 1913, Pre-Commerce, Panama-Pacific File, HHP, HHPL.

23. Hoover to Moore, August 20, 1913, Pre-Commerce, Panama-Pacific File, HHP, HHPL.

24. Hoover to John Barneson, September 4, 1913, Pre-Commerce, Panama-Pacific File, HHP, HHPL.

25. *Who's Who, 1914* (London, 1915), pp. 321-22.

26. Hoover to W. A. M. Goode; Goode to Hoover, September 13, 1913, Pre-Commerce, Panama-Pacific File, HHP, HHPL.

27. Moore to Hoover, September 20, 1913, Pre-Commerce, Panama-Pacific File, HHP, HHPL.

28. Hoover to Moore, September 19, 1913, Pre-Commerce, Panama-Pacific File, HHP, HHPL.

29. Hoover to Barneson, September 4, 1913, Pre-Commerce, Panama-Pacific File, HHP, HHPL.

30. Hoover to Frederick Skiff, September 30, 1913, "Panama Pacific International Exposition, Miscellaneous, P-Z," Pre-Commerce, Panama-Pacific File, HHP, HHPL.

31. Hoover to Moore, October 13, 1913, Pre-Commerce, Panama-Pacific File, HHP, HHPL.

32. Skiff to Hoover, October 3, 1913, "Panama Pacific International Exposition, Miscellaneous, P-Z," Pre-Commerce, Panama-Pacific File, HHP, HHPL.

33. Hoover to Moore, September 30, 1913, Pre-Commerce, Panama-Pacific File, HHP, HHPL.

34. A copy of the memorandum to the government is reproduced on pages 43-45 of the British committee's pamphlet, *The Panama-Pacific Exposition: The Facts of the Case.*
T

35. Hoover to Moore, November 11, 1913, Pre-Commerce, Panama-Pacific File, HHP, HHPL.

36. Goode to Hoover, October 11, 1913, Pre-Commerce, Panama-Pacific File, HHP, HHPL.

37. *Who Was Who, 1916-1928,* p. 983.

38. On pages 11-42 of the committee's publicity pamphlet, *The Panama Pacific Exposition: The Facts of the Case,* dozens of favorable editorials from all over the United Kingdom are reprinted, thus indicating the extent of the press influence that Hoover and Goode achieved in the autumn and winter of 1913-14.

39. Goode to Hoover, October 14, 1913, Pre-Commerce, Panama-Pacific File, HHP, HHPL.

40. Hoover to Moore, October 19, 1913, Pre-Commerce, Panama-Pacific File, HHP, HHPL.

41. Goode to Hoover, November 24, 1913, Pre-Commerce, Panama-Pacific File, HHP, HHPL.

42. Hoover to Moore, November 25, 1913, Pre-Commerce, Panama-Pacific File, HHP, HHPL.

43. Hoover to Moore, November 17, 1913, Pre-Commerce, Panama-Pacific File, HHP, HHPL.

44. Hoover to Barneson, December 5, 1913, Pre-Commerce, Panama-Pacific File, HHP, HHPL.

45. Hoover to Moore, December 5, 1913, Pre-Commerce, Panama-Pacific File, HHP, HHPL.

46. Hoover to Moore, December 6, 1913, Pre-Commerce, Panama-Pacific File, HHP, HHPL.

47. Goode to Hoover, December 19, 1913, Pre-Commerce, Panama-Pacific File, HHP, HHPL.

48.   Goode to Hoover, January 2, 1914; Hoover to Goode, January 6, 1914, Pre-Commerce, Panama-Pacific File, HHP, HHPL.

49.   Victoria Allen, "The Outside Man," 1:145-46.

50.   Confronted with widespread labor and feminist unrest and the very real threat of treason in the army and in sections of the Conservative party over the issue of Irish independence, the Liberal government was apparently simply too overwhelmed with crises to reconsider the Exposition question in the spring of 1914 in spite of majority sentiment in the House of Commons (George Dangerfield, *The Strange Death of Liberal England, 1910-1914*, pp. 333-401). British entry into World War I, of course, ended any lingering hopes that Britain might participate. Considering the political situation in England, Hoover could well be pleased with his work.

Hoover's fleeting reference to the Panama-Pacific episode in his *Memoirs* shows that he eventually came to believe that the government actually did reverse its decision not to participate as a result of pressure "at the needed spot—the House of Commons" (Hoover, *Memoirs*, 1:120).

3 The Club of Public Opinion and the War

WHEN HERBERT HOOVER entered public life in 1914 as chairman of the Commission for Relief in Belgium, his experience in the Panama-Pacific Exposition affair stood him in good stead. Public relations promptly became a key factor in the success of that organization; and subsequently, it would become crucial in his activities as food administrator and head of the American Relief Administration. In all of these organizations, Hoover preferred to work through the mass media and numerous subordinates, while he himself remained largely in the background. As in the case of his work with the Stanford student government and the Exposition, he saw himself and acted as a hidden catalyst "stimulating others to action." What had worked before was now applied on a grand scale; and it was during the war period that his characteristic administrative style achieved maturity and the foundations were laid for his later application of a behind-the-scenes, public relations approach to American social and economic problems.

I

When the outbreak of hostilities occurred in August, 1914, Hoover, as we have seen, was in London serving the interests of the Exposition; and it was there that the chain of events carrying him into "the slippery road of public life," as he later put it, was set in motion.[1] Several days after the war began, he had created an impromptu organization to attend to the monetary needs of stranded

American tourists, people whose traveler's checks, because of the panic created by the war, were not being honored by British banks, hotels, or restaurants. In connection with this American Committee in London, he had also organized, through engineering associates, an American Refugee Committee in Brussels, which enabled stranded Americans on the Continent to make their way to London. On this committee was Millard Shaler, who, late in September, 1914, informed Hoover that the food supplies he had purchased for famine-threatened Brussels were being held in England by the British government—the British being apprehensive that the food would fall into the hands of the German army. Hoover carried Shaler's problem to American Ambassador Walter Hines Page, and the latter, through informal discussions with Foreign Minister Edward Grey, was able to secure free passage of the food with the understanding that no further shipments would be permitted. Hoover then consulted with his friend Melville E. Stone, general manager of the Associated Press, who also happened to be in London at the time. Cognizant of the potential usefulness of American public opinion even at this early date, he suggested that Stone "ventilate the tragic plight of the Belgians and Northern France in America." At the time, Hoover planned to leave for the United States in late October, but before his sailing date arrived, Ambassador Page and other American and Belgian diplomats and businessmen, greatly impressed with the young engineer's administrative ability and international experience, were pressing him to head a permanent organization for the relief of the Belgians. On October 19, he made the momentous decision to accept the chairmanship of the Commission for Relief in Belgium.[2]

With Shaler's experience fresh in his mind, Hoover realized at the outset that success was dependent upon the organization of a "great campaign for charity the world over not only to secure funds but to create a world opinion that would keep the door to Belgium open through the [British] blockade and keep the Germans from taking food from [the Belgians]."[3] He thus turned instinctively to his friends in the mass media, men upon whom he could depend in his efforts to solicit the needed funds and apply the "wide propaganda of newspaper publicity."[4] Edgar Rickard, the man who had introduced him to Millard Shaler, was his original choice for handling publicity.[5] However, when Rickard soon took on other assignments within the organization, Hoover solicited the assistance of another London companion with press connections, Associated Press correspondent Ben S. Allen. Allen broke off negotiations through which he and Hoover were seeking to purchase the Sacramento *Union* and came quickly to Europe to publicize the Belgian cause from the commission's London office. With the permission of Melville Stone, he sent almost daily dispatches via the A. P. wire, "Strong punch[es] of cable from [the] scene of action," as Hoover called them.[6] In his early releases, the first of hundreds he would issue over a five-year period, he reiterated to the American public the desperateness of the Belgian food situation, described the organization of the CRB and the steps already taken by it to provide relief, and called for the consolidation of all independent Belgian relief committees into the centralized structure of the CRB.[7] Will Irwin, "the best press agent in [the] world" in Hoover's eyes, and at the time a war correspondent for the *Saturday Evening Post*, also answered Hoover's call for help.[8] Returning to America, where he headed the press department of the commission's New York office, he prepared daily and weekly news releases to papers and press associations, composed pamphlets and handbooks for the use of local commission committees, and wrote copy for the free advertising that the commission received in both magazines and newspapers.[9]

Through these publicity efforts, the CRB was placed on a firm footing in the United States. But its success elsewhere was by no means assured. In January, 1915, the British renewed their threats of a blockade, claiming that, just as they had feared initially, the food supplies to Belgium were passing into the hands of the German military authorities. They were thus aiding the German war machine rather than providing succor to the people,[10] and unless the CRB could guarantee effective food controls that would prevent this, they intended to allow no further shipments. To meet this challenge, Hoover again sought to mobilize the power of the press. Before setting off for Berlin to negotiate with the German government, he cabled Secretary of State William Jennings Bryan, asking him to discuss the situation with the German ambassador in Washington in an "influential way," to emphasize that, if present practices continued, the moral responsibility for the decimation of the population would be laid at the German door, and to impress upon the Germans the inadvisability of having "these issues tried in the court of American public opinion."[11] To supplement this line of attack, he also had Allen dispatch a lengthy statement to the American press from the CRB office in London, one designed to place further pressure on the German government. After describing the precarious situation of the Belgians, the release concluded: "If all fails, the neutral world and future generations will lay the responsibility for the decimation of these people at the proper door, and no mixture of military reason and diplomatic excuse will cloud the issue. . . . We have stated our case bluntly and frankly. Our only court of appeal is American public opinion, and it is for America to say whether a crime shall be committed which will bring this generation down in infamy."[12]

Through such methods, Hoover, in his own words, prepared a "club of public opinion,"[13] and once he began negotiating, this did prove effective. He was able to secure assurances from the Germans that they would "stop all taking of food from Belgium and Northern France," assurances "confirmed in writing through [American] Ambassador [to Germany James W.] Gerard and generally carried out."[14] He was also able to secure increased British financial assistance for the work of the CRB. In doing so, he invited Chancellor of the Exchequer David Lloyd-George to consider the consequences for Britain of an inflamed "public sentiment in the United States."[15]

In the summer of 1915, Hoover raised the "club of public opinion" over the head of a new threat to the CRB's work, a threat now originating from within the United States. Senator Henry Cabot Lodge of Massachusetts, so Hoover learned, was making investigations and formulating an attack upon him for alleged violations of the Logan Act, a law dating back to the 1790s, which prohibited negotiations between American citizens and foreign governments. Since in Hoover's mind "the maintenance of public confidence and good will in the United States was the very life-blood of our work," and since "in the hands of a sensational press," Lodge's activities "might do irreparable injury among neutrals, and give a weapon to the militarist groups in Britain and Germany [with which] to attack" the CRB,[16] he moved quickly to thwart them. Arriving in New York in May, 1915, he again sought the assistance of his friend, Melville Stone, the influential general manager of the Associated Press. The latter quickly arranged for a dinner, attended by the leading New York editors and publishers and by the heads of the other press agencies; and at this, Hoover received assurances that these men would use their journals to counteract any charges Lodge might make. In addition, to further buttress his position, he persuaded President Wilson to issue a press release from the White House, commending the CRB's work and listing the names of important leaders from the business world who were supporting it—"men whose backgrounds could not be challenged."[17] Thus fortified, he then confronted Lodge personally, meeting with him in Boston and coming away certain that the senator had been "misinformed" and "that nothing would happen."[18] Once again he had used the press and the friendship of journalists to protect the CRB from a potentially harmful action.

Consequently, by the summer of 1915, the CRB was operating efficiently in Belgium, unhampered by the combatants. Keeping it in operation, however, meant that Hoover must maintain a steady flow of American charity funds to supplement the subsidies of the British, French, and Belgian governments; and in securing these, he could not continue indefinitely to invoke the image of a starving Belgian nation without undermining the credibility of the whole organization and running the risk of a complete cessation of American aid. The situation seemed to call for a change of tactics, and in devising one, Hoover took his cue from his former press agent for the Panama-Pacific campaign, William Goode. The latter, after being enlisted to raise funds in England and throughout the British Empire, had achieved great results through the committee method of organization and publicity. In Hoover's view, he had become "far and away the most successful man" of all those engaged in organizing private relief.[19] And it was to

Goode's committee techniques that the CRB now turned. In August, 1915, its chairman decided that in America further appeals for the relief of Belgium would be carried out under the aegis of local committees established throughout the country.[20]

Hoover's view of the matter was set forth in a particularly explicit letter to Lindon W. Bates, an old engineering associate whom Hoover had made head of the commission's New York office. In it, Hoover reveals much about his sensitivity to the role and limitations of the press in forming public opinion, and also indicates his early appreciation of how a decentralized, local committee structure, a device upon which he would rely heavily throughout his public career, could be used to carry out public policies:

> It appears to me, from the considerable experience which we have now had in all phases of this work, that certain features have developed. We initially appealed for foodstuffs for a starving nation, but we have since built up an economic machine by which this is no longer a legitimate undercurrent of appeal and we have long since abandoned it everywhere except that these phases of the matter seem to crop up in the American mind. The only legitimate, honest appeal which we have the right to make to the public now is for food, money, or clothing for the *destitute* in Belgium. Any other basis of appeal is subject to refutation at once as dishonest, and must lead us into criticism. Furthermore, in the initial stages in order to bring vividly before the world the right of the Belgians to import foodstuffs, we engaged in a wide propaganda of newspaper publicity. This material had great news value and was freely used and in the main served to create a public opinion in support of the Commission's objects. This phase is now firmly established, and the material no longer has news value and is no longer received by the press. Practically, the era of publicity in the daily prodding of the newspaper is entirely over and is degenerating into personal puffs. It is a useless waste of money, time, and energy to pursue it, and lacks dignity appropos the position we have arrived at. . . .[21]

For Hoover, the "only real[ly] fruitful method" for soliciting benevolence now lay in "strong decentralized community organization."[22] In the initial weeks of the CRB's existence, he himself had telegraphed governors and influential friends urging the establishment of state collecting committees. Will Irwin's press campaign out of the New York office had, in fact, been designed to bring in contributions to these committees.[23] Now, however, in light of Goode's remarkable success, he was prepared to rely almost exclusively upon committee organization, for, as he continued in his letter to Bates:

> The thing which produces money and material is the personal interest and solicitation of people of standing in each community. Practically our most successful field to date has been the Australasian Colonies where we have issued but one document and that was originally an appeal from the London office. The whole of the work has been done by closely knit and able local committees and has produced so far practically as much money out of the five millions of people as has been produced out of the whole ninety millions in the United States. Likewise the organization in England of a special general committee with subcommittees in every locality has produced extraordinarily gratifying results with the use of scarcely any newspaper publicity, and even this has been accomplished in competition with a thousand other funds which are in the field. . . . In other words, the whole of this is to show that the effective result is obtained practically by supplying material to the committees only, at least from now on. When one comes to the question of committee organization, we immediately come to the question of personal *amour propre*. In order to gain the best results, one has got to elevate the efforts of the individuals in these committees to as high a point as is possible in order to give them a stimulating interest which is absolutely necessary.[24]

True to the sentiments expressed in this letter, Hoover, for the balance of his tenure as chairman of the CRB, concentrated upon organizing and using local committees in carrying out relief campaigns. During the winter of 1915–16, under the inspiration of a moving directive, his newly formed committees undertook a widespread campaign for the collection of clothing; and in 1916 and 1917, as a special supplement to the overall effort, they emphasized the theme of children's relief.[25] To bolster the work of these committees, Hoover was able to secure the assistance of George Barr

Baker, a former newspaperman and magazine editor, who, early in 1916, began service as a Hoover public relations aide that would run through the presidential years.[26] Replacing Will Irwin, who had returned to "cover the front" for the *Saturday Evening Post*, Baker supported the committee collection work out of the commission's New York office by "planting" favorable publicity in the daily and periodical press and lining up the support of prestigious individuals and institutions.[27] Enthusiastic public endorsements, material assistance, and a willingness to cooperate were elicited from former President Roosevelt, the Federal Council of Churches, the Rockefeller Foundation, and the Daughters of the American Revolution.[28] But Baker's greatest public relations coup was scored in October, 1916, when he traveled to Rome, bearing a plea to Pope Benedict XV to issue a statement supporting the children's drive. The pope, once chary of taking any action that might be construed as political, now responded positively by authorizing the American Catholic clergy to solicit funds and send them on to the CRB.[29]

By 1917, Hoover had created a far-flung public relations apparatus. Through newspaper and magazine publicity, the instigation of specialized sub-campaigns at the community and state level, and the association of important public figures and renowned institutions with his work, he had been successful in securing the material and moral support necessary to bring Belgium safely through her period of national travail. Working through his friends in the press and through the thousands of committees organized at his urging, he had "wielded the club of public opinion" and achieved gratifyingly concrete results—notably, the raising of nearly one billion dollars for the purchase and shipment of over five million tons of food and clothing.[30] Accordingly, in the spring of 1917, when American entry into World War I created the need for food conservation within the United States, his experience and his high standing in the eyes of Ambassador Page and Colonel Edward M. House, both trusted advisers of President Wilson, made him the logical choice for food administrator. From London he moved to Washington and thus inaugurated the American phase of his public career.[31]

II

As food administrator, Hoover was responsible for securing American food surpluses and seeing that they reached the citizens and troops of the Allied powers. His task, in other words, was no longer the simple humanitarian one of feeding starving people; it was now inextricably linked to winning the war. And already, some months before he accepted the appointment, he had given considerable thought to the administrative methods he would use and the large role that public relations would play. In an interview with Will Irwin, he had drawn upon his firsthand observation of British mobilization, reflected on his own experience with the CRB, and noted:

> Much can be done by national propaganda to limit extravagance in eating, dress, and display. The British tried that. With their energies taxed in every direction, they hadn't time to give the matter much attention or energy. The propaganda went no further than influencing the newspapers, putting out a poster or so, and encouraging discussion. Even at that it accomplished a great deal. We could give much more energy to this matter by a central bureau in Washington, with subcommittees all over the United States. That is one place where we could use our women to great advantage. We are good advertisers. A few phrases, too, would turn the trick—and the world lives by phrases, and we most of all perhaps. . . . We need some phrase that puts the stamp of shame on wasteful eating, dressing, and display of jewelry. . . . We could not bring the law to bear on this, only educate and direct public opinion.[32]

In his new post, Hoover would put these random thoughts into action. Public relations techniques would again play a key role, much as they had for the CRB; and within what he referred to as his "theory of administration," publicity would function as a link between the "centralized ideas" of his Washington office and the "decentralized execution" of those ideas by state food administration officials, by women, and by the public at large.[33]

As in the case of the CRB, too, Hoover's first efforts to "educate and direct public opinion" took the form of securing the assistance of the press and using it to carry the food conservation message to the American people. Again he prevailed upon Melville Stone, this time to allow Ben Allen to sever completely his ties with the Associated Press and take over what would variously be called the Department of the Press, Division of Public Information, Publicity Division, and finally, to avoid confusion with the Creel Committee on Public Information, the Education Division of the Food Administration.[34] And again, shortly after organizing this division, he sent a letter to 2,500 members of the press, explaining his purposes and appealing for their cooperation. "The world as a whole," he noted, was "faced with a definite and growing food shortage" that would have an "important bearing on our national life, not only as affecting our task of supporting our allies in the war, but in its ultimate reactions upon our entire range of food industries and the life of our people." He recognized that in dealing with an "intelligent people," it was necessary to prove "the case that such a shortage exists . . . and that . . . proof must be furnished as a basis for creating the dominant idea in the national mind that we must enlarge our food service to the world, not only as a war measure, but as a measure of humanity itself." If he could "secure the emplacement of this idea in the minds of the people, the sequent suggestions of constructive order" that he might make would "fall not only on a receptive mind but upon a convinced intelligence." To secure the "awakening of the national conscience and to guide the public mind in [the] channels" of food conservation, he realized that he was "wholly and absolutely dependent upon the press of the country." If he did not receive its support, "the problem [was] hopeless." If he had it, "it [could] be solved."[35]

Once he had made his personal appeal, Hoover also demonstrated in his dealings with the press that, from the governmental side, he meant to extend full cooperation and make available all information concerning the operations of his organization. Avoiding the "censorship bugbear" that soured relations between the Creel Committee and the reporters,[36] he guaranteed complete access to the news, and by doing so, was able to establish warm and cordial ties with newsmen, ties that remained strong until his presidency. In response, for example, to their desire for personal contacts, he appeared at weekly press conferences, and when there was information of unusual importance, on unscheduled occasions as well.[37] And having secured friendly relations, he exploited them to the limit, allowing the press to play a major role in his operations.

In all, from May, 1917, to April, 1919, Hoover "reached out to the public" through 1,870 press releases, some 1,400 of them prepared by Allen's staff and dispatched to the Washington press corps, and an additional 470 directed at the rural press and particular regions and issued through the offices of the state food administrators. By means of these hundreds of releases, the Food Administration kept the American people informed of its purposes and goals, instructed them in new ways to save food, and advised them of the progress being made.[38] It also employed the same techniques to put "the stamp of shame" on individuals who were not cooperating or were found in violation of the Lever Act, the law under which the food controls were now operating. Some thirty releases exposed to public scrutiny the names of entrepreneurs and companies whose operations had been closed, suspended, or fined for infractions of the law.[39] Nor was this all. In addition to their educational and punitive functions, the releases served as stimulants to action. True to his conviction that "the world lives by phrases, and we most of all," Hoover used his Education Division to proliferate hundreds of exhortatory slogans and "patriotic fillers" (e.g., "Food Will Win the War," "Do Not Help the Hun at Meal Time") and to persuade editors to use them, both in editorial writing and for those "one, two, and three line places in the makeup."[40] Evidently, too, he felt such techniques were highly successful. After a year in office, Hoover was moved to comment that without "the absolute devotion and teamwork of every newspaper in the United States" he could not have attained his ends. "Every appeal through this gigantic influence," he noted, had been given "an immediate and prompt distribution."[41]

As chairman of the CBR, Hoover had also been impressed by the influence of such magazines as the *Literary Digest, Bookman, Collier's, Independent, Ladies' Home Journal, Outlook,* and *World's Work,* all of which had volunteered in support of his efforts.[42] Through such media, he had come to realize, contact could be made with people not necessarily reached by the daily press. And accordingly, as food administrator, he resolved to make greater and more systematic use of them. To do so, he subdivided the Education Division into sections serving periodicals with special clienteles. There was a section, for example, whose work was devoted solely to the woman's journals, another for the trade and labor journals, a third for the farm journals and country weeklies, a fourth for religious journals, and still another for the Negro press. Gertrude B. Lane, editor of the *Woman's Home Companion*, headed the woman's section, assuming, in Hoover's words, "the responsibility of establishing the connection, throughout existing avenues, between the women of the country and the Food Administration." James H. Collins, formerly a business journalist for the *Saturday Evening Post*, directed the trade and technical section, sending *Weekly Bulletins* to 1,500 trade journals, 350 labor journals, and 900 business house organs. A massive effort to reach the all-important farmer was launched on the pages of the farm journals and country weeklies by Charles W. Holman, a former editor and secretary of the National Conference on Marketing and Farm Credits. Howard B. Grose, editor of the Northern Baptist *Missions*, was assigned to send bulletins to 750 religious journals and 85,000 clergymen of all faiths, and Professor E. T. Attwell of Tuskegee Institute was appointed head of the Negro press section to "educate" Negroes on proper dietary habits and to thwart the attempts of German propagandists to undermine the loyalty of black Americans. A professional photographer, Mrs. Lloyd E. Allen, supplied all these people with photographs as director of the Section of Illustrations.[43] In the magazine field, as well as in that of newspapers, Hoover had shown himself to be highly adept at organizing all available "existing avenues" of communication.

However, notably in his work for the CRB, Hoover had come to feel that newspaper and magazine publicity could go only so far in stimulating interest and motivating public action. In addition to such publicity, there was the need for appealing to "personal *amour propre*," for elevating "the efforts of individuals to as high a point as is possible in order to give them a stimulating interest which is absolutely necessary." In particular, he hoped now that women could be involved and "used to great advantage," especially since they, as a group, "controlled at their own tables about 80 per cent of the nation's food consumption." Properly organized and motivated, they could be a great aid in his task; and consequently, he proceeded to embark on a massive public relations drive, designed to appeal to their desire for patriotic sacrifice and to give them a sense of participation.[44]

In the summer and autumn of 1917, he launched two separate "personal-pledge campaigns" in communities all across the country. In conducting these, he began by gathering field representatives in Washington and instructing them on the food situation at home and abroad. The representatives were then sent into each of the states to organize drives in the local communities. In the first effort, housewives were asked, either by a solicitor in person or through the mails, to sign cards pledging them, as members of the Food Administration, to carry out its requests in the conduct of their households. Those who signed and sent their pledges to Washington received two new cards, one to be displayed in their windows as an emblem of "membership," the other to be posted in the kitchen where its instructions on how to maximize food-saving would be a constant reminder to its holder. In the second campaign, some 500,000 canvassers, assisted by newspapers, churches, and schools, sought to enlist those who had not yet signed such pledges. Eventually, between thirteen and fourteen million families were recruited as active members of the Food Administration.[45] And through them, Hoover tried to control consumption so as to compensate for increased demands abroad and inadequate supplies at home. At his urging, special "wheatless," "meatless," and "porkless" days were officially proclaimed by President Wilson; and once these were established and highly publicized, both nationally and locally, the Food Administration could call upon its millions of "members" to observe them.[46] The result, Hoover later recalled, was "exactly what [he] expected—a wealth of co-operation" in the fight to eliminate domestic wasting of food.[47]

The public relations "pledge" campaign approach was also "perhaps the most important single agency relied upon to bring the wholesale and retail trades into complete cooperation with the Food Administration." This, at any rate, was the opinion of Albert Merritt, who in October, 1917, took charge of the publicity work of the Distribution Division.[48] Although the Lever Act authorized the use of legal sanctions against wholesalers, Hoover preferred, wherever possible, to gain their support through voluntary cooperation. And one way of doing this was through large "pledge posters," distributed by Merritt to all those licensed under the Lever Act. Such distributors were asked by Hoover himself to sign the pledge inscribed on the poster and display it, thus making them, like the individual households, "official members" of the Food Administration. These "members," moreover, were expected to use their salesmen to distribute Food Administration literature and to obtain similar pledges from retailers, a group not covered by the Lever Act.[49] The idea, as Hoover once put it, was to plaster "the hoardings of the country with posters."[50] And again, he did achieve gratifying results. In the grocery trade alone, some 25,000 traveling salesmen of the wholesale houses became directly involved and eventually distributed about 430,000 pledge posters.[51] As both Hoover and Merritt saw it, such "democratic [methods] of getting results, though slow," were the best ones, for after the emergency, the people would be "inspired by the knowledge that they had won by their own endeavor."[52]

As Merritt also notes, there was yet another way in which publicity was used to control the unlicensed food retailers. In the spring of 1918, the Food Administration established Price Interpreting Boards composed of wholesale grocers, retailers, and consumers. These boards, created in 1,200 counties and communities across the country, set "fair prices" for wholesalers and retailers. These were then published in local newspapers under the heading "Fair Prices for [   ] County," and those retailers not complying with the agreed-upon price standards could thus be easily brought into line by the threat of boycott, both from the wholesale distributor and from the consumer.[53]

In addition to extensive use of the press and the launching of pledge card, poster, and "fair price" campaigns, Hoover sought to reach the "public mind" through the "channels" provided by the infant but rapidly growing advertising and motion picture industries. In these fields, he apparently acted independently of the Committee on Public Information[54] and, in some respects, in advance of it. Mullendore, at any rate, credits the Food Administration with being the first war organization to utilize the "American genius for advertising."[55] Under the expert leadership of C. E. Raymond, vice-president of the J. Walter Thompson Company and "a pioneer of modern advertising," and R. C. Maxwell, president of his own billboard advertising firm,[56] it received an estimated nineteen million dollars of free advertising space, donated not only by outdoor (billboard) advertising firms but also by magazines, newspapers, railways, bus and streetcar companies, and muncipalities. It also enlisted the cooperation of the motion picture industry, particularly in the production of many short reels illustrating food conservation techniques in the home, films that were then distributed among colleges, schools, and social and civic organizations.[57]

Finally, a variety of social institutions, including the schools (from the elementary up through the collegiate ranks), the churches, the libraries, and the patriotic, fraternal, and religious societies, were likewise engaged in the campaign for food conservation.[58] Through numerous conferences and through the employment by Hoover of special personnel functioning as liaison between the Food Administration and these institutions, they, too, were induced to sign pledges of cooperation and, once enlisted, were provided with thousands of bulletins and pamphlets, explaining what they could do to save food and how they could persuade others to cooperate.[59]

In Hoover's mind, moreover, this whole approach was a great success. Citing Department of Agriculture statistics, he maintained that the net export of foodstuffs in 1917-18 (15.1 million tons) had more than doubled, when compared with the average of the three years preceding American entry into the war (6.4 million tons). And in 1918-19, he argued, the export figure of 18.6 million tons represented nearly a tripling of the prewar average.[60] Much of this increase, to be sure, was due to greater crop production. Yet Hoover was convinced that his "education and direction" of public opinion had also greatly augmented the amounts of food shipped abroad and had enabled him to stabilize food prices without re-sorting to excessive governmental controls. The "thousand insistent appeals" made through newspapermen and advertisers, along with the "devotion of the great numbers of committees," had, he felt, "given an intimate understanding for each man, woman, and child in the United States of the objectives of government," and by do-ing so, had "solved the problem" of food conservation without ra-tioning and at a minimum cost in public funds.[61]

III

With the coming of the Armistice in November, 1918, Hoover's procurement of food for Europe and the public relations accom-panying this effort did not come to an end. Even before the ces-sation of hostilities, he had understood that the continued shipment of American food supplies to postwar Europe would be necessary to prevent famine there, and, having made his concern known to President Wilson, had been requested on November 7, 1918, "to undertake the transformation of the Food Administration into [a] new agency of relief and reconstruction [in Europe]."[62] The new agency, the American Relief Administration, was funded by a $100,000,000 Congressional appropriation and, under Hoover's di-rection, helped feed Europe's needy during the period of peace negotiations at Versailles. However, all official United States relief work ended in June, 1919, with the signing of the treaty.[63] Aware that hunger was still widespread—especially in central and eastern Europe, Hoover secured the president's approval "to transform the public organization into a private one which would continue the work under the same [ARA] title."[64] To raise the funds necessary to purchase and distribute food, he returned to the public relations and organizational tactics that had proven so successful with the CRB and the Food Administration.

From the summer of 1919 through the summer of 1921, Hoover organized and served as chairman for two distinct private relief campaigns, both based on the compelling theme of preventing the starvation of the children of Europe. The first, running through the European harvest of 1920, was directed by an agency entitled the A.R.A. European Children's Fund. Edgar Rickard and Gertrude Lane served on the ECF's executive committee and publicized the fund-raising efforts of state committees created by the reactivation of old CRB and Food Administration personnel. Meanwhile, George Barr Baker, fresh from service as a naval communications censor, rejoined Hoover in Paris to handle the ECF's overseas publicity arrangements.[65] Hoover had originally estimated that American charity would be required only through the summer of 1920. Nevertheless, massive crop failures soon made obvious the need for a second and more sweeping appeal to the American public.

In the summer of 1920, then, he laid the foundation for a huge collection to be undertaken by a body called the European Relief Council, a federated organization, chaired by himself and consisting of the ARA, the Red Cross, the Friends Service Committee, the Jewish Joint Distribution Committee, the Federal Council of Churches, the Knights of Columbus, the YMCA, and the YWCA.[66] Again, the structure of the ERC consisted of statewide committees established under the auspices of a prestigious central committee composed of representatives of the cooperating groups. To help the committee reach the collection goal of $33,000,000 deemed necessary to save an estimated three and one-half million starving children,[67] Hoover placed Baker in charge of conducting the council's public relations. Installed in an office at 42 Broadway in New York City, Baker solicited public endorsements from President Wilson, President-elect Harding, and, once again, from Pope Benedict XV. Assisted by the public relations firm Lupton A. Wilkinson, Inc., he prepared vividly entitled pamphlets (e.g., "Shall It Be Life or Death?"), advertisements, articles, and special appeals to the clergy, which were then distributed to the press and magazines on a nationwide basis. For local dissemination, he sent these same materials to the state publicity directors. Instructional bulletins designed to coordinate the activities of the local committees with those of Hoover as national chairman also passed from Baker to the state leaders at regular intervals during the winter of 1920-21.[68]

Baker's work, however, was not limited simply to propaganda placed in the printed media. He put together a motion picture, "Starvation," based on film made by the ARA in Russia, which was shown frequently in New York City. To insure wide reporting and viewing of the movie, he sent free tickets to influential New Yorkers including editors of the newspapers, magazines, and trade journals.[69] He dispatched mica slides "to every motion picture house in the United States" and urged chairmen to see that they were in fact shown by the local theater managers.[70] To dramatize the collection even further, he and Hoover inaugurated in December, 1920, a series of banquets in honor of the "Invisible Guest," i.e., the needy European child, who was symbolized in the dining hall by a lighted candle at the center of the head table. At these intensively publicized banquets, which Hoover recalled as "one of our most useful ideas," wealthy Americans paid one thousand dollars to eat relief rations and thus contribute to the salvation of the "waifs and orphans" of Europe.[71] Though the drive closed in March, 1921, some three million dollars short of its goal,[72] Hoover could well regard the effort as a success—especially since it had been carried out after a prolonged period of sacrifice and in a time of economic recession.[73]

IV

In terms of his future career in the executive branch of the government, the significance of Hoover's wartime public relations activities can hardly be overstated. The creation of newspaper publicity by such press agents as Ben Allen and George Barr Baker, the tactical use of the press release at crucial moments, the cultivation of good relationships with newspaper and magazine editors and reporters, the involvement achieved by "pledges" and posters, and the appeals made through local committees involving hundreds of individuals—all of these techniques were merely amplifications of the methods Hoover had employed in his prewar fight for the Panama-Pacific Exposition. But where the Exposition tactics had ended with indifferent (though not disappointing) results, there could be no mistaking, in Hoover's eyes, the achievements of similar tactics deployed on a much larger scale during the war years. The success of these devices in mobilizing public support for national policies was not lost upon him, and it was only natural that he should turn to them in his next administrative assignment, that of secretary of commerce. Before discussing how he employed them in the 1920s, however, it is necessary to describe the public relations apparatus he built for that purpose and also to examine closely his personal and intellectual motives for doing so.

1. Herbert Hoover, *The Memoirs of Herbert Hoover, 1874-1920: Years of Adventure,* 1:148.

2. Ibid., pp. 152-56.

3. Ibid., p. 155.

4. George I. Gay, with the collaboration of H. H. Fisher, *Public Relations of the Commission for Relief in Belgium,* 2:269.

5. Ibid., 1:16-17.

6. Ibid., 2:240, 256.

7. Ibid., pp. 239-43; "Publicity and Press Reports of the C.R.B., 1914-1919," Hoover Institution on War, Revolution, and Peace, Stanford, Calif.

8. Gay and Fisher, *Public Relations of the Commission for Relief in Belgium,* 2:256.

9. Ibid., pp. 245-46.

10. Hoover, *Memoirs,* 1:162.

11. Gay and Fisher, *Public Relations of the Commission for Relief in Belgium,* 1:236-37.

12. Ibid., pp. 237-40.

13. Victoria Allen, "The Outside Man," (unpublished, undated), 2:166, Ben Allen Papers, Herbert Hoover Presidential Library; Will Irwin, *Herbert Hoover: A Reminiscent Biography,* p. 175.

14. Hoover, *Memoirs,* 1:165-66.

15. Gay and Fisher, *Public Relations of the Commission for Relief in Belgium,* 1:263-66.

16. Hoover, *Memoirs,* 1:199-201.

17. Ibid., p. 200.

18. Ibid.

19. Gay and Fisher, *Public Relations of the Commission for Relief in Belgium,* 2:270.

20. Ibid.

21. Ibid., pp. 268-69.

22.   Ibid.

23.   Ibid., pp. 247-52.

24.   Ibid., pp. 269-70.

25.   Ibid., pp. 270-78.

26.   George Barr Baker, "The Great Fat Fight," pp. 12-13.

27.   George Barr Baker Papers, "Goode, William A.," Hoover Institution on War, Revolution, and Peace.

28.   Gay and Fisher, *Public Relations of the Commission for Relief in Belgium,* 2:271-72, 281-82.

29.   Baker to William Goode, October 13, 1916; Baker to W. B. Poland, November 3, 1916, George Barr Baker Papers, "Goode, William A.," and "Poland, W. B.," Hoover Institution on War, Revolution, and Peace; Baker, "The Pope and the 'Lone Crusader,'" pp. 16-17; Gay and Fisher, *Public Relations of the Commission for Relief in Belgium,* 2:277-80.

30.   Gay and Fisher, *Public Relations of the Commission for Relief in Belgium,* 2:182-83.

31.   Irwin, *Herbert Hoover,* pp. 187-88; Hoover, *Memoirs,* 1:199, 212-15, 218-20, 225.

32.   Hoover made this statement during an interview with Will Irwin for the *Saturday Evening Post.* In the article, Hoover's identity is masked behind the pseudonym "Smith" (Irwin, "First Aid to America," *Saturday Evening Post,* March 24, 1917, 1-B, Public Statements, HHP, HHPL).

33.   Evidently impressed with the success of the decentralized structure of the CRB, Hoover determined at the outset of his work with the Food Administration to decentralize its operations through the creation of state food administrations. In a statement of June 19, 1917, before the Senate Committee on Agriculture, he spoke of "the erection in every State of the Union . . . [of] some form of food administration and the decentralization of our functions so far as possible into the State administrations. . . . It is our desire to decentralize our administration into the hands of the State administrations at every point possible. Our theory of administration is that we should centralize ideas and decentralize execution" (William C. Mullendore, *The History of the United States Food Administration,* p. 70).

34.   Allen, "The Outside Man," 4:399-400; Maxcy R. Dickson, *The Food Front in World War I* (Washington, 1944), pp. 25-26.

35.   Quoted in Mullendore, *The History of the United States Food Administration,* p. 83.

36.   George Creel, *How We Advertised America,* pp. 16-27.

37.   Mullendore, *The History of the United States Food Administration,* p. 84. The Washington press corps was so appreciative of Hoover's attentive concern for their work that on July 8, 1918, they paid him an unusual tribute. In a signed statement they "saluted" him "as an official who has made good." In their eyes, he had "played the part [of Food Administrator] well." He had "stood the test" (Press tribute to Hoover, July 8, 1918, Food Administration Files, HHP, HHPL). For two students of the press and government during the war, the newspapermen performed their duties in what "was practically a partnership with Hoover" (Minna Lewinson and Henry B. Hough, *A History of Services Rendered to the Public by the American Press During the Year 1917* [New York, 1918], p. 15).

38.   "Press Releases," Food Administration Files, Hoover Papers; Mullendore, *The History of the United States Food Administration,* 84. At the state level, the

state food administrators were also active in establishing ties with state and local news media. Education Divisions were often created within the state organizations. See for instance, Ivan L. Pollock, *The Food Administration in Iowa*, I, especially, chapter 4.

39. "Press Releases Index," Food Administration Files, HHP, HHPL.

40. "Press Releases," Food Administration Files, HHP, HHPL.

41. Hoover, "Pittsburgh Press Club Address," April, 1918, 7-C, Public Statements, HHP, HHPL.

42. Gay and Fisher, *The Public Relations of the Commission for Relief in Belgium*, 2:245.

43. Mullendore, *The History of the United States Food Administration*, p. 85; Dickson, *The Food Front in World War I*, pp. 28-30; Food Administration Files, "Edgar Rickard, Personnel," Box 32, Hoover Institution on War, Revolution, and Peace.

44. Herbert Hoover, *An American Epic*, 2:57.

45. Mullendore, *The History of the United States Food Administration*, pp. 86-87; Dickson, *The Food Front in World War I*, pp. 138-39.

46. Dickson, *The Food Front in World War I*, pp. 142-43; Hoover, *An American Epic*, 2:60-62.

47. Hoover, *Memoirs*, 1:250.

48. Albert N. Merritt, *War Time Control of Distribution of Foods*, pp. 53, 214.

49. Ibid., pp. 53-54.

50. Hoover, "Pittsburgh Press Club Address."

51. Merritt, *War Time Control*, p. 54.

52. Quoted from publicity brochure, "Enlisting the Food Merchant" in Merritt, *War Time Control*, pp. 59-60.

53. Ibid., pp. 110-12.

54. Creel, *How We Advertised America*, pp. 156-65, 273-82. In general, it appears from Creel's account and from Mullendore's history that the public relations activities of the two organizations were set up independently and operated with little coordination.

55. *The History of the United States Food Administration*, p. 88.

56. Food Administration Files, "Edgar Rickard, Personnel," Box 32, Hoover Institution on War, Revolution, and Peace; Dickson, *The Food Front in World War I*, p. 31.

57. Dickson, *The Food Front in World War I*, pp. 90-95; Food Administration Files, Herbert Hoover Archives, "Education Division, Moving Pictures," Hoover Institution on War, Revolution, and Peace.

58. Mullendore, *The History of the United States Food Administration*, pp. 90-95.

59. Ibid.; Edith Guerrier, *We Pledged Allegiance: A Librarian's Intimate Story of the United States Food Administration*, pp. 78-101; *The Food Front in World War I*, pp. 86-91, 114-19.

60. Hoover, *Memoirs*, 1:270.

61. Ibid., Hoover, "Pittsburgh Press Club Address"; "Address to St. Louis Advertising Club," October 12, 1920, 94, Public Statements, HHP, HHPL.

62. Hoover, *Memoirs*, 1:276.

63.   Frank M. Surface and Raymond L. Bland, *American Food in the World War and Reconstruction Period*, p. 5.

64.   Ibid., p. 6; Hoover, *Memoirs*, 2:18.

65.   Hoover, *Memoirs*, 2:18-19; Edgar Rickard to Hoover, May 29, 1919, Food Administration Files, "Personnel," Box 32; Baker to A.R.A. Personnel Officer, June 7, 1919, George Barr Baker Papers, "A.R.A. Miscellaneous," Box 9, Hoover Institution on War, Revolution, and Peace; "U.S. Naval Censorship Executive Finishing Fine War Record," *Editor and Publisher* 52 (September 11, 1919): 20.

66.   Hoover, *Memoirs*, 2:20-21.

67.   The ratio between the monetary goal and the number of children to be saved evidently suggested to Hoover the fund-raising slogan, "Ten dollars will save a child," which was used in all the ERC's propaganda materials (Hoover, "Organization of Child Relief in Europe," n.d., American Relief Administration Papers, "A.R.—82," Hoover Institution on War, Revolution, and Peace).

68.   Lupton A. Wilkinson, "Feeding Hungry Europe," *Current History* 13 (November, 1920): 322-24; American Relief Administration Papers, "A.R.—23," to "A.R.—82," especially Baker's memorandum to state chairmen, "Publicity Supplies," December 13, 1920, A.R.—36, Hoover Institution on War, Revolution, and Peace.

69.   George Barr Baker Papers, "Motion Pictures," Box 12, Hoover Institution on War, Revolution, and Peace.

70.   Memorandum, Baker to State Chairmen, "Publicity Supplies," December 13, 1920.

71.   Hoover, *An American Epic*, 3:256-58; Telegram, Hoover to State Chairmen, December 17-18, 1920, "Preparation of Invisible Guest Certificate," American Relief Administration Papers, "A.R.—40," Hoover Institution on War, Revolution, and Peace.

72.   In a memorandum analyzing the problems encountered during the collection, Edgar Rickard noted that the *Literary Digest*, desiring to make a "scoop," had incorrectly announced that the council's goal had been attained. He thus blamed the failure to reach the $33 million mark on the lack of "absolute control of publicity" during the campaign (Rickard, "European Relief Council: Confidential Summary of the National Collection," n.d., Edward Eyre Hunt Collection, "American Relief Administration, C.R.B.," Box 2, Hoover Institution on War, Revolution, and Peace).

73.   Surface and Bland, *American Food in the World War and Reconstruction Period*, p. 79.

4 An Outside Influence

By 1921, HERBERT HOOVER, because of his great penchant for administrative publicity, had created a web of connections with the mass media of communications of truly remarkable dimensions. As secretary of commerce from 1921 through 1928, his public relations personnel and ties with the press continued to proliferate —so much so, in fact, that by 1928 he was perhaps the most heralded public official in the country. By that time, even though he was opposed by the political professionals, his renown and "grass roots" strength were so great that he was an unstoppable candidate for the Republican nomination and then for the presidency of the United States itself.

As one examines during this period Hoover's burgeoning public relations apparatus and his ties with the press, three questions naturally arise. One concerns the men involved and the techniques they used. The second concerns the formation of his press connections and the role that they played in his administrative style. The third, long a highly debated one, concerns motivation. Did he, in other words, consciously mobilize public relations around his activities in order to serve presidential ambitions? The present chapter will consider each of these questions and will offer, in particular, some conclusions about motives and ambitions as suggested by a further analysis of his "enigmatic" personality and his attitudes toward "personal publicity."

I

One of the most popular and respected public men in America, Hoover was named secretary of commerce by President Warren

G. Harding in March, 1921. He was convinced, as always, that his department's "usefulness to the country" was "dependent solely upon its ability to get information to the country,"[1] and for this reason, he took pains in his new work to reestablish the close ties with the press that had been a hallmark of his earlier administrations. For some reason, perhaps his greater appreciation of the work of George Barr Baker and Edgar Rickard, he had ended his relationship with his longtime press assistant, Ben Allen.[2] For a man of Hoover's stature, however, finding competent press assistants to replace Allen proved no problem. While retaining Baker and Rickard to finish old projects and begin new ones in New York City,[3] he was able to build around him a team of new men in Washington, a truly remarkable group with wide newspaper and magazine experience, who would manage his expanded press relations and publicity needs as secretary of commerce.

There was, for example, Christian A. Herter, who would become editor of *Independent* and *Sportsman's* magazines in 1924 and, much later, a congressman and governor of Massachusetts and secretary of state under President Dwight D. Eisenhower. As secretary to American Peace Commissioner Henry White, Herter had become acquainted with Hoover at the Peace Conference in Paris. He had then done some secretarial and publicity work for Hoover's European relief projects in the period from 1919 to 1921. Now he became Hoover's initial press "assistant" in Washington.[4] Following Herter, there was Harold Phelps Stokes, a veteran reporter for the New York *Evening Post* and Washington *Evening Post*, who served Hoover from 1924 to 1926. As with Herter, Stokes had evidently become acquainted with, and devoted to, Hoover at the Paris Peace Conference.[5] When he left the Commerce Department to join the editorial staff of the New York *Times*, Stokes was succeeded by George Akerson, a friend of Hoover's since 1921 as Washington correspondent for the Minneapolis *Tribune*. A key figure in publicizing Hoover's candidacy for the Republican nomination in 1928, Akerson remained with Hoover as his press secretary into the third year of his presidency.[6]

Herter, Stokes, and Akerson, with their extensive ties to the daily and periodical press and their devotion to their "Chief," provided excellent liaison between the Commerce Department and the public. In addition to the traditional secretarial chores, it was their job to scan the pages of the daily press in order to answer any criticisms or correct pieces of misinformation concerning the department. They also frequently responded to requests from fellow newsmen, known to them on a first-name basis, for information about Hoover's work. Paid by Hoover personally, since an economy-minded Congress refused to appropriate money to increase the department's staff,[7] these three "private assistants," as Hoover called them, may well have been unprecedented figures in the service of a cabinet officer. Certainly, such press secretaries had never been found before in the Commerce Department.[8]

But Herter, Stokes, and Akerson were only a few of the "scribes" whom Hoover called to his side in his efforts to interpret his work to the American public. Another key figure, for instance, was Edward Eyre Hunt, who had been an editor of *American Magazine*, a war correspondent, an American CRB official in Antwerp, and one of the first writers to bring Hoover's work in Belgium before the American public. His attractive literary portrait of Hoover in his book *War Bread: A Personal Narrative of the War and Relief in Belgium* (1916) was reproduced in the *New Republic* in September, 1916, and in the *World's Work* of June, 1917. In this sketch, Hunt had prophesied that "the public service of Herbert Clark Hoover has just begun. He belongs not only to Belgium but to America, and as soon as the war is over and Belgium is free, his own country will have need of him."[9] His prophecy had come true, and, in 1920, Hunt himself had become secretary and publicist for Hoover's committee on the Elimination of Waste in Industry. Following the completion of this task, he remained with Hoover as a quasi public relations man, working as secretary or member of a number of Hoover-initiated projects, among them the Conference on Unemployment in 1921; the United States Coal Commission in 1922-23; the study of Recent Economic Changes in 1928; the President's Committee on Recent Social Trends in 1930; the President's Emergency Committee for Employment in 1930-31; and the World Economic Depression Inquiry in 1931.[10] Most of these conferences, committees, and commissions produced reports of their findings, and it was Hunt's responsibility to give them continuity and prepare them for publication—a job usually handled by the McGraw-Hill Company, with which Hunt and Hoover had especially close ties.

From 1921 through 1924, Hunt published some eight statements of varying length commenting upon various aspects of Hoover's work as secretary of commerce. The pieces appeared in the *Outlook, Survey,* and the *Nation.* In 1924, in his introduction to a set of essays published in a volume entitled *Scientific Management Since Taylor,* he further celebrated Hoover as instrumental in bringing the principles of Frederick W. Taylor's "scientific management" to fruition on the level of national government.[11] In short, Hunt functioned as a medium transmitting Hoover's "liberal industrial program," as he called it, to the American public. He had envisioned the elimination of waste in industry report as merely the "thin point of the wedge," "the opening gun" of Hoover's campaign for public education on sound industrial policies. Deeply impressed with Hoover's "ability to advance action . . . along with public education," he remained a key publicist for the administrator through his presidential years.[12]

Two other important figures, men who also helped Hoover to communicate his programs to the American people and, more specifically, to the business community, were Archibald W. Shaw and Frederick Feiker. Arch Shaw was an industrial editor and publisher who worked closely with Hoover throughout his Commerce Department years. Chairman of the Conservation Division of the War Industries Board, a position in which he had first become acquainted with Hoover, Shaw had returned after the war to the management of his Chicago publishing house, which issued the well-known industrial journals *Factory Magazine* and *System Magazine,* the latter with a circulation of over a half-million.[13] In March, 1921, Hoover offered Shaw the position of assistant secretary of commerce, and though Shaw declined, he did agree to spend extended periods of time in Washington helping Hoover reorganize the department, secure needed appropriations, and develop his simplification program for industry. In April, 1922, Shaw again declined Hoover's request that he become assistant secretary, but he continued to serve Hoover from his publisher's desk. Editorials and articles describing and praising the secretary's work appeared frequently in the pages of *Factory* and *System*— as did Hoover's own statements and those of his many assistants.[14]

But perhaps Shaw's greatest service to Hoover lay in securing for him the talents of his good friend Frederick Feiker. Feiker had been a technical journalist with the General Electric Company, the editor of *Factory*, chairman of the editorial board of *System*, and editor of *Electrical World*. When, at Shaw's urging, he came to Hoover's side in May, 1921, he was a vice-president of McGraw Hill Company in charge of sixteen technical and industrial journals that it published.[15] Feeling that he could help in putting "constructive forces" to work molding "public opinion along broad lines of business policy,"[16] he arranged for a six-month leave and became Hoover's full-time aide. When the latter was impressed with his "extraordinary piece of work," Feiker stayed on for another three months, helping "the business papers of the country," as James McGraw put it, to do "their full duty in interpreting government, and particularly the Department of Commerce . . . , to industry."[17]

In addition to helping Edward Hunt in his effort to make Mc-Graw-Hill *the* "publishing house willing to take up [Hoover's industrial] program and push it hard,"[18] Feiker also labored to establish close ties between Hoover and other major components of the business press. Only a month after assuming office, he arranged for the secretary to meet with business press editors representing some fifty-six industries, a meeting at which Hoover promised further consultation in the future and asked the conferees to make known to their readers the ways in which the department and business could cooperate in serving each other's needs.[19] And even after he had left the department, Feiker continued to serve Hoover by advertising his work in McGraw's trade periodicals and other magazines, printing statements of his publicity aides, arranging further conferences with the business press editors, and giving advice on how the meetings might be made even more profitable.[20] Hoover, for his part, found the work of the editors of "utmost importance in bettering the organization of the Department."[21] He saw to it that they were well supplied with material covering the department's activities,[22] and they, in turn, were appreciative. At the 1924 annual meeting of the Associated Business Papers, Inc., the editors commended Hoover for the "recognition which he has accorded the business press" and pledged their "whole-hearted cooperation,"[23] something that became even closer when Feiker himself became their managing director in 1927. Once more he assured Hoover of his support. "When I see you," he wrote, "I should like to talk with you about the possibilities of this organization of some one hundred and twenty-four business and technical publications reaching 1,110,270 men in industry and trade."[24]

Still another figure in the Hoover public relations group, one who also deserves special mention, was Donald Wilhelm, a veteran magazine writer specializing in political and economic subjects, whose work in Washington dated back to Theodore Roosevelt's administration. During the war, Wilhelm had become interested in government publicity work and had written excitedly of the way in which both the Creel Committee on Public Information and the Food Administration under Hoover had succeeded in their attempts at "Americanization," i.e., in "making the entire country conversant with the spirit of the United States at war."[25] A great admirer of Hoover, he had celebrated him during the war and then helped "boom" him for the presidency, notably in interviews and articles for the *Independent* and the *Review of Reviews*.[26] In April, 1921, he wrote Hoover, saying that he would feel "greatly honored if there should be any way in which, in my rather humble field, I could lend a hand at any time." In January, 1922, Hoover assigned him to the department's staff, where he remained throughout the year, receiving his pay partly out of the funds of the Bureau of Standards ($4,500) and partly out of Hoover's own pocket ($1,500).[27]

Wilhelm's major job was to secure magazine publicity for the Bureau of Standards, whose work was being overshadowed by the massive publicity campaign already being carried out in behalf of the Bureau of Foreign and Domestic Commerce. Over the years, he had contributed dozens of articles to most of the major American magazines, had come to know their editors and staffs personally, and was therefore ideally suited for establishing the necessary contacts. Within a few weeks of his appointment, he reported enthusiastically to Feiker:

> The *World's Work* has my article on the Department—just in time to do the most good on the Hill [in getting appropriations].
> The *Illustrated World* is soon to publish an article of mine on the Housing Division.
> *Forbes' Magazine* is soon to publish one on the trade associations and their helpfulness to the Department.
> Herbert Corey did an article for his syndicate of Associated Newspapers—a thousand strong. I got him and filled him up. Paul Kellogg, of the *Survey*, whom I wrote, sent down Miss [Adele] Shaw. I have *Collier's* interested; likewise *Leslie's* and the *Outlook*. The *Saturday Evening Post* is on the job, through Kenneth Roberts.
> B. C. Forbes, who edits *Forbes' Magazine* and reaches papers all over the world through the Phila[delphia] *Ledger Syndicate*, is coming down. Rene Bache, who writes a science page every week for the same syndicate, is in touch, waiting with his mouth open for anything I can feed him from the Bureau [of Standards]. As soon as I can get squared off, I can 'feed' *Illustrated World*, *Popular Science*, and *Popular Mechanics* in the same way. . . .[28]

A week or so later, Wilhelm notified Hoover in another memorandum that he had arranged for articles on the department's and the Bureau of Standards' work with Roberts and Albert Atwood of the *Saturday Evening Post*, with Miss Shaw and John Ihlder of the *Survey*, with William M. Houghton and Samuel Hopkins Adams of *Leslie's Weekly*, with Merle Thorpe of the *Nation's Business*, and with Albert Shaw of the *Review of Reviews*.[29] All of these editors and reporters had been invited to tour the various bureaus of the department in order to gather material for articles, which, in most cases, duly appeared in their journals. Beyond this, Wilhem also prodded government scientists in the bureau's radio and aviation sections to write articles, which he then arranged to have published in popular, and not simply, technical periodicals.

In addition, special research documents emanating from the Bureau of Standards on subjects such as radio, aviation, and measurements were publicized in advance by press releases sent to newspapers across the country. Wilhelm was convinced that the releases—"describing in a page or two [and] in a very popular way what the publication is about"—"enormously increased the usefulness of the document." By such means, as he himself put it, he dug "the Bureau of Standards out of the snow."[30]

In the course of his year's publicity work for the Department of Commerce, Wilhelm did not neglect its secretary either. Working closely with his good friend French Strother, the editor of *World's Work*, he prepared an article for the magazine's February issue entitled, "Mr. Hoover as Secretary of Commerce: What He Has Done to Make His Department a Real Aid to Commercial Development."[31] When Senator Wesley Jones, chairman of the Senate Commerce Committee and member of the Senate Appropriations Committee, requested in January, 1922, that Hoover give him some material that might assist him in procuring appropriations for the department, Hoover had Wilhelm send him the manuscript of his article along with other information. Wilhelm reported to Hoover that Jones had found the material "exactly what he wanted" and that it was being sent to the Republican National Committee for general distribution to all Republican Senators and Congressmen—though, as in the case of the published *World's Work* article, the information "was not marked as coming from this office."[32] It was also the indefatigable Wilhelm who "discovered" Hoover's little essay "American Individualism," and who arranged, again in collaboration with Strother, to have it appear as an article in the April, 1922, *World's Work* and then, later in the year, in book form with Doubleday, Page, and Company.[33]

Paul J. Croghan was still another important cog in Hoover's Department of Commerce publicity machinery. He was unique among the secretary's publicists in that he was a holdover in the department from the previous administration. Under William C. Redfield and J. W. Alexander, President Wilson's secretaries of commerce, Croghan had operated a press service related entirely to the welfare of the Bureau of Foreign and Domestic Commerce.

In a memorandum to Feiker of May, 1921, concerning the establishment of publicity for the department, Croghan noted that it had become "evident some years ago that if we [the Bureau of Foreign and Domestic Commerce] were to survive [i.e., receive appropriations], it was essential that the Bureau's work be advertised and friendly relations established with the almighty press."[34] Such relations, though, had never been very extensive.

It was not until the coming of Hoover that Croghan's "press service," under the urging and direction of Feiker,[35] became a dynamic "Press Bureau" serving the whole Commerce Department. From it, newspapermen received steady streams of Hoover's addresses, his frequent statements on matters of topical concern, and material, such as Wilhelm worked up for the Bureau of Standards, designed to arouse the public interest in the thousands of reports published by the department. Croghan commented in a memorandum to Stokes that in 1925 alone some 2,000 hours of overtime were logged by the Mimeograph Division of his bureau, i.e., "2000 after office hours were necessary by from five to twenty employees of this Division to perform some job from the Secretary's Office."[36] In fact, so much news poured out of the Commerce Department during Hoover's years that David Lawrence, in setting up the *United States Daily,* a journal designed to cover the federal government, anticipated that he would need three reporters to handle Hoover's department alone: one for the Bureau of Foreign and Domestic Commerce, one for the Bureau of Standards, and one for the other bureaus of the department. To the presidential office and the other departments of the executive branch, he felt he would have to assign only one or, in the case of the Department of Agriculture, two correspondents.[37]

Croghan was also important in arranging well-attended press conferences that Hoover presided over at regular intervals in his office.[38] Through such cultivation of the press, the secretary came to be viewed as one of the best sources of news in Washington. As Croghan noted to Herter in a memorandum of August, 1921: "The Department is now considered by newspaper men generally as the one real source of news in the city. Just the other day the Washington *Star* man told me that 'Hoover certainly has got the whole town by the neck from a news standpoint.' From the talk that comes in to me daily, I am sure this is the general feeling."[39] Although naturally subject to self-interested exaggeration, Croghan's judgment here is corroborated in the reminiscences of several Washington correspondents. Leo Rosten has recalled that "Herbert Hoover welcomed newspapermen to his office and discussed national affairs with them frankly and informally. The press corps felt that he was the best 'grapevine' in Washington." Remembering the same period, Herbert Corey has written that Hoover "was unquestionably the favorite of the Washington correspondents during this time, for as the head of a department he could spare time to get acquainted with them. The representative correspondents called on him, got his views on what was going on here and everywhere else, and relied upon his judgment and his perfect candor." In Corey's view, "no other public man in Washington was ever more thoroughly known to the newspapermen whose job it is to watch all public men, or more highly respected by them."[40]

Of course, Hoover did have a few editorial adversaries, and among these none was more important than the powerful William Randolph Hearst, who disliked Hoover for his favoring of the United States entry into the League of Nations and for his alleged anglophilism. But here again, through the efforts of men like Croghan and Shaw, the secretary of commerce was able to secure a "good press" even in the Hearst papers. In 1924, for instance, Hoover asked Shaw "to set straight" George Hinman, a Hearst reporter, on a Department of Commerce policy. Shaw was able to report success on his mission. A year later, Croghan reported:

> Letters like the attached from Meloon, Financial Editor of the Boston *American* [a Hearst paper], the most remarkable editorial support we have received repeatedly from Hinman; the thousands of dollars worth of free space which men like Thornburgh of the I.N.S. [Hearst's International News Service] gladly provide right along, seem to point to the fact that while Hearst himself may not be favorable to this Department, his attitude is not reflected in the output of the men he employs. . . .
> We have made a special effort for the last three years to give extra good service to Hearst representatives and I think our

efforts in this direction are at least partly responsible for their apparent very friendly attitude towards us at this time.[41]

In addition to these activities, Croghan worked closely with Julius Klein, director of the Bureau of Foreign and Domestic Commerce, to publicize Hoover's trade expansion program. Within a year after Hoover assumed office, he had persuaded scores of newspapers across the United States to subscribe to a special weekly "Department of Commerce page,"[42] surveying economic conditions and advertising "trade opportunities." The page was written by two bureau trade commissioners with newspaper experience, men who had been recalled from their posts in Australia and China for this express purpose, and it did seem to be especially well received.[43] As Croghan reported to Klein in the spring of 1922, Leo Sacks of the Scripps-McRae Press Service had signed up thirty-two of his papers and had commented to him that "the Department of Commerce news service [was] the best in town bar none."[44] For the first time, too, he was succeeding in placing Commerce Department news in southern newspapers and in the foreign language press.[45] In all, he and Klein liked to boast, of the 5,000,000 readers of the subscribed newspapers, two million read the commercial news made available by the Commerce Department.[46]

Also integrally related to Hoover's publicity scheme as secretary of commerce was the Lupton A. Wilkinson public relations firm, headquartered in New York City, but with branches in Boston, Chicago, San Francisco, Atlanta, and Washington, D.C. Hoover employed Wilkinson to supplement the work of Croghan in the department's press bureau and that of Herter (and later Stokes) out of his own office. Again, too, old connections were important. Wilkinson and his vice-president, Raymond C. Mayer, had collaborated with George Barr Baker in the publicizing of Hoover's European relief projects; and consequently, when Hoover joined the cabinet, they were promptly retained by him to keep a newspaper clipping service designed to gauge the effectiveness of his publicity and keep abreast of editorial reactions. Along with this, they also prepared press releases for Croghan, composed magazine articles discussing Hoover's programs, and wrote the synoptic prefixes to the secretary's addresses that were frequently sent to newspapers. These summarizations, as Wilkinson wrote Hoover, were designed "to sell the importance of the speech to correspondents and editors at a glance. We hope of course that your fuller summarization will be used in each instance, but no harm can possibly be done by co-presentation of the shorter one. This kind of service to the press never results in less space; always in more."[47]

The incorporation of Lupton Wilkinson's services into the Department of Commerce public relations apparatus was a manifestation of Hoover's conviction that, as he put it, "public relations —publicity and advertising—[had] become an exact science"[48] and indispensable to government administration. Actually it might be noted here, he himself had been one of the first conscious experimenters with "public relations" on a large scale, for he had long practiced (since 1912 and 1913, in fact) the very techniques that "pioneers" in the field such as Edward Bernays were codifying in the early 1920s as a new "science." As we have seen, Hoover had not only "wielded the club of public opinion" through the mobilization of the press and the use of the well-publicized slogan, but also had had recourse to a variety of public relations "stunts" such as the "pledge cards" and "wheatless" and "meatless" days of the Food Administration and the "invisible guest" banquets of the ARA period. Given the parallel rise of his publicity-oriented career with that of the "public relations industry" itself, it was natural that a man like Bernays would be in frequent contact with him.[49] It is also understandable that John Lee Mahin, president of the Federal Advertising Agency of New York City, might observe to Hoover that "the recent talk I had with you tended to deepen an impression which I have had for some time—that your publicity work was probably as important a feature of your work as any other phase of it."[50] In addition to Bernays and Mahin, Hoover also had access, through George Barr Baker, to the informal counsel of New York's other leading public relations figures, among them the famed Ivy Lee whom Baker, a good friend, termed "the leading publicist in America."[51]

One operation that well illustrated Hoover's public relations machine and approach in action was that of preparing and publicizing the secretary's *Annual Report* to the president. Required by law to account for money spent and to describe work undertaken during the preceding fiscal year, Hoover viewed the 1922 *Report*, his first full *Report* as secretary of commerce, as an opportunity for getting across "the idea" that his secretaryship was "revolutionary—something new" in the department's history.[52] Under Redfield, the *Annual Reports* had been rather matter-of-fact descriptions of the department's work; but now they were intended to stress the fact that under "vigorous reorganization" the department had become "a real Department of Commerce . . . responding to the needs of the business world," that "it was bigger, more competent, and more successful" than ever before.[53] Hoover gave special instructions to Wilkinson, Croghan, Baker, and Herter to lay out a plan for such a report. To create a demand for its appearance, he ordered appropriate parts of it released to the trade journals and to the local chapters of the Chamber of Commerce, an organization that was now headed by his old friend and subordinate in the Food Administration, Julius Barnes.[54] This practice was also continued after 1922. In subsequent years, Hoover instructed his staff to have sections of the *Report*, pertaining to specific bureaus and divisions, released on a staggered, one-a-day basis during the week immediately preceding the publication of the full report.[55]

In addition, Hoover insured the widest possible circulation of his *Reports* by distributing literally thousands more of them than had his predecessor. Redfield had sent out about 1,000 copies to the president, the cabinet, Congress, and interested manufacturers and newsmen. In 1922, along with this "regular distribution," Hoover disseminated over 11,000 additional copies. They went to the presidents and secretaries of chambers of commerce (2,564), to trade associations (2,525), to railroad and coal companies (1,084), to governors and mayors (688), to trade and agricultural journals (1,850), to members of the department's five advisory committees (1,159), and to numerous miscellaneous recipients (1,500). And since the government permitted the free distribution of only 5,000 of them, Hoover paid for the balance printed, some 9,000, out of his own pocket, which, at a cost of 25c per copy, amounted to $2,250.[56] In subsequent years, copies were not sent to the chambers of commerce, mayors, or trade associations, thus reducing the total number considerably, but Hoover saw to it that large numbers continued to reach the press. In 1923, for instance, over 5,000 copies were sent to the three major press associations (the Associated Press, the United Press, and the International News Service) and to trade and agricultural journals; and even though the press services prepared their own summaries, Croghan also had a summary statement that was sent out "to every paper reached by the associations."[57] If at all possible, it seemed, Hoover was determined to impress upon the public the fact that, where two years earlier the Commerce Department had been "the tenth Department of government in influence and service," it had come under his guidance to rank "among the first three with the Treasury and State Departments in its constructive influence upon national welfare."[58]

II

Thanks to the efforts of publicists such as Herter, Hunt, Shaw, Feiker, Wilhelm, Croghan, and Wilkinson, "the constructive influence" of the secretary of commerce was indeed quickly "impressed upon the public." But vast as Hoover's public relations were, it should be realized that the great and growing renown of the administrator was by no means simply a product of paid propagandists as has been frequently charged. To appreciate fully the magnitude of the publicity attending the man and his work as secretary of commerce, it is necessary to indicate at this point the depth and extent of the good will freely accorded to Hoover by the fourth estate and the reasons for it.

As chairman of the CRB and as food administrator, Hoover had received much unsolicited publicity because of the compelling nature of his work.[59] His efforts in Belgium, after all, had been crucial to the survival of millions of people, and those as food administrator had been inseparable from the task of winning the war by sacrificing "on the home front." In both tasks, moreover, he had been eminently successful, a fact that made him the recipient of much favorable publicity at the war's end. Widely perceived as the embodiment of "practical idealism," as both the "Quaker humanitarian" and "efficient engineer," a combination of great symbolic potency in the United States of 1920, he was celebrated by the press as the man best suited to guide America's fortunes through the social and economic wreckage of the postwar world.[60] The "Hoover boom" for the presidency in 1920, stoked as it was by newspaper and magazine writers, derived in large part from the press's appreciation of Hoover's work and character and from the contemporary public appeal that these had, not from any deliberate "image creation" by press agents working on his behalf.

Consequently, when Hoover became secretary of commerce, he continued to reap the benefits of favorable publicity from writers and editors who had eagerly supported him earlier and who did not need to be "cultivated" by his public relations men. Such influential editors of mass circulation magazines as George Lorimer of the *Saturday Evening Post*, Norman Hapgood of *Hearst's International Magazine*, and French Strother of *World's Work* had all been ardent promoters of Hoover for the presidency in the period 1919-20. In November, 1919, Lorimer had written a three-column editorial calling for the American people to eschew professors and lawyers and choose a businessman with a thorough knowledge of the economy for their next president,[61] and though he named no names, he was pleased that of the many readers responding favorably, all mentioned Hoover's name. Subsequently, he had Will Irwin, then writing for the *Post*, do an article on Hoover,[62] and in April and November, 1920, Hoover himself published lengthy articles in Lorimer's magazine.[63] Hapgood had also been captivated by Hoover's war work. Having become a personal friend of Hoover's during the war, he had represented Hoover's position in an April, 1920, conference with the editors of the New York *World* and the *New Republic* who were going "to talk out their future attitude" toward Hoover.[64] Strother, as noted above, had contributed to the "Hoover boom" with a lengthy elaboration of his experience and qualifications for the presidency. Though they failed to get their man in the White House, these men rallied to his side as secretary of commerce—viewing him as the most important executive officer on domestic affairs in national government. They wholeheartedly shared the attitude of Hartford Powel, editor of *Collier's* and yet another influential Hoover advocate, who wrote Hoover in November, 1921, that he was "ready to be of any possible service to you or to your Department."[65]

Hapgood, Strother, and Powel, helpful to Hoover though they were, could not compete with Lorimer in this regard. Lorimer's great esteem for Hoover produced much free "press agenting" from *Post* reporters such as Isaac Marcosson, Garrett Garet, and Samuel Blythe. All these men became good friends and skillful advertisers of Hoover and his work. Marcosson, in particular, was of value to Hoover in his 1926 serialized account of the Commerce Department's trade expansion program. Bearing Hoover's personal request to department trade commissioners abroad that he receive all "courtesy" and "assistance" in collecting materials for his stories, Marcosson toured the world in order to be able to dramatize the "adventures in exotic lands" of men whose work spurred American foreign trade.[66] In 1926, he had his articles published in book form with that "old and distinguished house," Harpers. He dedicated the book to Hoover, put his picture on the frontispiece, and entitled the work, *Caravans of Commerce*, a title, he felt, that would bring "color, romance, and book store appeal" to the work while avoiding "the suggestion of a technical trade hand-book."[67]

Ever ready to supply department material to the *Post* writers, who asked for it frequently on a wide variety of matters, Hoover was also able to exploit his warm relationship with Lorimer to have matters of personal concern aired in the magazine. A remarkable instance of this occurred in the spring of 1923, when Hoover wrote Lorimer requesting that he print a piece "on the personality and work of President Harding," whom, he felt, had been "misrepresented" as a "weakling" and "golf-playing" president "when as a matter of fact he works like a slave."[68] When Lorimer proved willing to go along, Hoover arranged an interview between the president and Samuel Blythe;[69] and the result was Blythe's July 28, 1923, article ("undertaken without any initiative save my own")

"A Calm View of a Calm Man," which praised Harding as the right man for the times.[70] Similarly, in 1927, Hoover was "moved to suggest" that he himself "write a piece about the Mississippi flood" because he had "a sort of intimate knowledge of this river . . . that might enable me to say something that would be entertaining to your readers."[71] Lorimer again approved the request, but Hoover never did get around to writing the story—though he continued to contemplate "taking advantage of your columns to illuminate the minds of the American people on the whole subject of our water resources from some new points of view."[72]

As in the case of Lorimer and his staff, then, much news concerning Hoover and his work as secretary of commerce resulted, not from the exertions of his public relations men but, rather, from friendships that he had established over the years with editors and writers. Hoover enjoyed these friendships with such influential journalists and editors as Edward Lowry, Hamilton Holt, William Allen White, Arthur Capper, Mark Sullivan, William Hard, Frederick Wile, Richard Oulahan, David Lawrence, Ida Tarbell, and Gertrude B. Lane. In his moments of relaxation and leisure, he had long enjoyed the company and acquaintances of writers, and the writers, in turn, found in Hoover a man of remarkably extensive knowledge of national and international affairs who was capable of enlivening his penetrating discussions of weighty issues with charming anecdotes and a subtle sense of humor. Such personal characteristics, plus the importance of the work Hoover was doing, explain why so many men of the press came to work for him so eagerly, and why so many others—such as those mentioned above—saw fit to publicize his work so favorably.[73] With this coterie of influential friends, Hoover also traded favors. He and his many assistants in the department supplied them with copies of his speeches, fed them information for their stories, articles, and books, allowed them special interviews, and enabled them to view as insiders the operations of his department, both in Washington and in the trade commissions abroad. In return, they gave wide circulation to his speeches and statements, both in print and on radio, arranged for him to meet and talk with special groups of editors and writers, defended him from occasional press attacks, and, in their own widely read articles concerning Hoover, lionized his abilities and achievements.[74]

III

Given the large number of publicists surrounding Hoover's work, it is understandable that several students of governmental publicity have looked upon him as instrumental in bringing the techniques of administrative publicity to maturity in American government.[75] And when one adds to the outpourings of his press bureau his friendly and productive associations with influential journalists, it is easy to see why his activities provoked suspicion that he was bent on advertising himself. As food administrator and in his first year as secretary of commerce, a few journalists, definitely a minority, came to feel that Hoover was employing "press agents" and "cultivating" relations with editors and reporters in order to create a public image of "miracle man," which would carry him to the White House,[76] and it was this type of suspicion that became accepted as fact for many writers during his depression-plagued presidency. But to what extent, if any, was Hoover actually bent on advertising himself? Can it truly be said that he deliberately created mass publicity for himself in order to become president of the United States? It is to these important and controversial questions that I shall now turn.

It was observed in the first two chapters that Hoover was temperamentally unsuited for public speaking and for offering a dramatic personal leadership even though he had been extremely influential in Stanford student government and in the overseas affairs of the Panama-Pacific Exposition. He abhorred public exposure of any sort, preferring to do his work through "front men" who carried out his policies. Closely guarding his personal privacy, he had achieved wealth and prestige in Stanford and mining circles while remaining unknown to virtually all but a few close friends and associates. When he became a "public man" in 1914, this passion for anonymity did not diminish, and this fact gives the lie to Hoover's legion of detractors during the depression who viewed his whole career as an exercise in self-promotion. For though Hoover habitually mobilized publicity around his work, he genuinely tried to keep his name out of it throughout his career. Self-advertising was manifestly not his aim, indeed, it was anathema to him. This self-effacing quality, in addition to the virtues attached to his organizational genius, helps explain why so many able men from all walks of life served their "Chief" so loyally and so unstintingly as subordinates. It is yet another reason why so many men of the press, both officially and informally, respected Hoover and were so willing to assist him in his wide-ranging endeavors.

Both as chairman of the CRB and as food administrator, Hoover labored studiously to maintain his anonymity. "We are only a group of glorified office boys," he told Ben Allen in 1914, "trying to get away with a tremendous job, and no individual has any right to get any glory out of it."[77] So desirous was he of keeping his name out of print that he dispatched his first press appeal for Belgium—one he had composed himself—over the name of Millard Shaler.[78] And Allen, in sending out his initial press releases under Hoover's name instead of under the name of the Commission for Relief in Belgium, disobeyed Hoover's explicit instructions and incurred his wrath. Only after a prolonged struggle was Allen able to secure his acquiescence in the use of his name. The extraction of a single photograph from him for publicity purposes was equally difficult. " 'Oh, how I wish the Chief would endure the limelight with more grace, but how I do admire him for disliking it,' " was Allen's frequent lament to his wife.[79] When Hoover, in spite of himself, became widely known for his CRB work, he was compelled to write in the May, 1917, *National Geographic Magazine*: "I always feel an infinite embarrassment at the reception and overestimation of the part that I may have played in what is really an institutional engine, and the credit for which belongs not to myself, but to some fifty thousand volunteers who have worked for a period of nearly three years."[80]

As food administrator, his attitude had been similar. In an interview published in July, 1917, he had "asked the press representatives not to personalize the Food Administration." He was aware that the American people had "a perfect mania for personalizing everything," but the Food Administration was "not personal." It would be composed of "probably several hundred of the best men that can be chosen in the country." He was therefore anxious that "if the [Food] administration [was] set up by the President after Congressional action, [his] own personality [should be] submerged in [the] institution and [his] own name disappear in the press." Publicity should be conducted "simply [for] the Food Administration."[81] Edward Bok, who as editor of the *Ladies' Home Journal* was a principal supporter of the publicity efforts of both the CRB and the Food Administration, wrestled with Hoover, as had Allen, over his attitude. In October, 1917, Bok was moved to write Hoover urging him "to put your personality forward. . . . There is a vast difference between what is said by the Food Administration and what is said by Herbert Hoover. The women believe in you, and they will follow a personal word from you where they overlook anything signed by the [Food] Administration."[82] Yet, Hoover continued to balk at the use of his name. A perusal of the hundreds of press releases emanating from Food Administration headquarters between 1917 and 1919 reveals that his name was mentioned only in a small fraction of them, primarily those containing his own statements.[83]

In his first few years as secretary of commerce, Hoover's scrupulous regard for avoiding self-advertisement lapsed somewhat—as evidenced by his instructions to his publicists concerning the *Annual Report* of 1922 and of 1923. But for the most part, his predominant concern was for publicizing the Department of Commerce as a whole, for, as William Hard has rightly said, "At bottom, Hoover [was] intensely an 'organization man.' "[84] In a December, 1921, letter to an editor who had recently subscribed to the department's "weekly page," Hoover expressed his views concerning the "institution" and the "individual":

I hope you will permit me to offer one suggestion as requested in your recent letter. It concerns the descriptive box which you use in advertising the Department of Commerce page. If it would not interfere with your plans too seriously, I would much prefer to have my name omitted—emphasis being placed on the

Department of Commerce as the source of the information rather than myself. It seems to me that constantly improving permanent service of government agencies must be built around the agencies themselves and not the temporary individual who happens on the job. To personalize it will, I fear, in the long run cause loss of interest in the many men who really do the work [and] to whom the Department and not the Secretary must be the inspiration of effort.[85]

On several other occasions, too, Hoover ordered Croghan not to use his name in press releases, except where the subject matter directly related to him;[86] and he once scolded Croghan for material approaching "too nearly the category of press agenting" and instructed him "to discourage extravagant popular treatment of any activity of the Department."[87]

No small part of the personal publicity concerning Hoover originated with his old friends from Stanford days—Will Irwin and Vernon Kellogg. Yet even these men—and other very close friends—who wrote of him in books and articles did so apprehensive of the fact that they might anger him by offending his sense of discretion. Kellogg inscribed a copy of his 1920 biography of Hoover: "To the victim with all commiserations."[88] And Will Irwin, in notifying Hoover of his forthcoming article in the *Post*, "Hoover as an Executive," wrote him: "I'm writing . . . trying to use my best judgment in discriminating between what is decent to print and what isn't. . . . Forgive much [*sic*] if I have to write you up and be thankful it is done by a friendly hand."[89] Donald Wilhelm also remembered some years after his work with Hoover had ended, that Hoover hated " 'personal stuff,' as he told me when there appeared in a weekly magazine an article about him that many public men would gladly have mortgaged their homes to get published about themselves."[90] On one of Wilhelm's own pieces, sent to the secretary for his approval, Hoover had written: "Please kill this. I want no personal advertising."[91] And still another old associate of Hoover, Alfred P. Dennis, prefaced his June, 1925, *Saturday Evening Post* article, "Humanizing the Department of Commerce," by noting that Hoover had commanded him "not to bring my personality into it." This was difficult, Dennis complained, "since his personality is infused through the Department from top to bottom." Merely noting this fact, he feared, was "risking a bad half hour with Mr. Hoover later on."[92]

In light of the evidence presented above, Hoover must be exonerated from the charge that he deliberately used public relations techniques to publicize himself. But what of the allegation that he was ambitious for the presidency even before 1920 and that, though perhaps discreet about it, he organized vast amounts of publicity around institutions he administered with the intention of boosting himself into the White House? Correspondence and other evidence at the Hoover Presidential Library and Hoover Institution discredit this view. Hoover, it appears, was never "bitten by the Presidential bee" and, even in 1928, can hardly be said to have run for the presidency. On the contrary, when taken in conjunction with Hoover's *Memoirs* and the autobiographical accounts of his friends, this evidence indicates that he "was run" for the office by the multitude of his former subordinates and admirers. For Hoover himself the kind of exposure that any really ambitious candidate for the presidency not only accepts, but enjoys, was thoroughly distasteful, and though extremely sensitive to criticism, he was also irritated by excessive public acclaim for his achievements. Hugh Gibson, an American diplomat in Brussels who had worked with Hoover in the CRB, was not exaggerating when he observed that Hoover "never suffers such acute misery as when being extolled publicly for what he has done."[93]

Typical of Hoover's attitude was his reaction in September, 1919, when, upon his return from Europe, he was besieged by letters from people urging him to accept the plaudits due him and to run for the presidency. His replies rejected both suggestions. To one correspondent, he wrote: "My ambition . . . is to get out of the limelight as fast as possible. . . . I do not like the notion of riding down the street with a band; and for all that I love the Star Spangled Banner and what it stands for I am just a little weary of standing at attention bareheaded in the sunshine or the rain, waiting for bands to massacre that sacred tune."[94] To another, he responded, "I am convinced that this country needs a few officials who will not be seeking for public honors for having done their simple duty."[95] To those who were interested in persuading him to run for the presidency, he was equally adamant:

> The whole idea fills my soul with complete revulsion. I want a rest and I need it. Any decent citizen is prepared to sacrifice himself and all his interests in a time of national emergency, but to enter into competition for the privilege of giving such a service, when there is no emergency, is a thing that I cannot bring myself to do. I do not believe it is a practical possibility, nor do I believe that I have the mental attitude or the politician's manner that is needed and, above all, I am too sensitive to political mud.[96]

When Caspar Hodgson, a Stanford classmate of Hoover and owner of World Book Publishers, observed to him in a letter that he could become President "if [you] would allow [your] friends to use the same publicity methods with which the question of food was gotten across to the American people," Hoover wrote back, "I cannot believe that I have the politician's skill needed to arrive at such a job."[97] And when Hodgson urged him as late as February, 1920, to respond to certain political attacks made upon him in a newspaper, Hoover replied, "I seem to get into the way of politically minded folks even when trying to keep out of politics."[98] A week later, he answered another friend:

> Consulting my own personal inclination I do not want public office. . . . You and your friends have urged that I should undertake to organize propaganda for myself, as representing issues, by entering into competition for nomination by a great party. . . . This implies entry upon a road of self-seeking, whereas my view is that I should agitate for issues, not for myself. . . . I am not so ignorant as not to realize perfectly well that such a course does not lead to nomination to the Presidency, but I would not be myself if I started out on a path of self-seeking to obtain my office.[99]

In late March, 1920, however, pressures on Hoover from close friends associated with his public service, especially those organized on his behalf in California, became so great that he finally made himself available for the Republican nomination. In a telegram sent to the head of the California group, Hoover stated: "While I do not and will not myself seek the nomination, if it is felt that the issues necessitate it and it is demanded of me I cannot refuse service."[100] True to his word, however, he steadfastly refused to campaign for the presidency. In an April 3, 1920, press release, he informed his supporters that his European relief work would prevent him from "taking part in a personal canvass." In the same release, he denounced those among his supporters who would ask him to place "partisanship above national interest," and he instructed others not to criticize rival candidates, for they [were] all "patriotic, honorable Americans . . . entitled to respect."[101] Lacking an avowed candidate, the Hoover movement of middle-class professional people—while gaining wide popular support—failed miserably in its efforts to achieve delegate strength. Hoover's lighthearted prophecy of March, 1920, that his "boom," like his son's "flivver," would take "a lot of people to start it," "make a lot of noise," and cause his supporters "to walk back home in the end," thus became self-fulfilling three months later at the Republican National Convention.[102]

One thing that the "Hoover boom" did produce, though, was the offer of a cabinet post, which the diffident administrator, though hesitant, found he could not refuse.[103] A cabinet position, especially the secretaryship of the Commerce Department, was, after all, ideally suited to Hoover's training and personality. In it, he could wield the influence over American social and economic issues that he had sought as early as 1907. Yet at the same time, it would enable him to work in the background, out of the "limelight," as was his wont. For several years, he apparently had been reconsidering an editorial career. Late in 1918, in making it clear to Edward M. House that he had no interest in the presidency, he had expressed his desire to buy an American newspaper and to "see what he could do with it."[104] In this same period, in dismissing the idea of the presidency, he had discussed in his correspondence the possibility of joining those "strong men," who might "with practically no organization, but with definite purpose, exert a greater influence on the [domestic and international] situation from the outside [rather] than from in."[105] And in 1919, he had, in fact, purchased shares in several newspapers, was managing one, negotiating for others,[106] and seemed, as we have seen, firmly convinced of the efficacy of the press in "educating and directing public opinion" and "illuminating the national mind." As in 1914, an editorial career may have appealed to him at this time as a means of achieving an "outside" and undemanding influence upon public affairs. But when the Commerce Department position opened up, this interest in newspaper management quickly abated. From this vantage point, he could exercise his need for self-assertion and satisfy his desire for influence in the shaping of policies. He might, given his contacts with writers and editors, exercise more power through the press as a cabinet officer than as editor of several newspapers. And he could work "behind the scenes," bearing none of the ultimate responsibility for decisions made or actions taken by the federal government.

One suspects, indeed, that Hoover's great desire for anonymity as chairman of the CRB and as food administrator had been something more than modesty, the legacy of his Quaker upbringing, or a concern for organizational morale. He had been quite anxious about assuming the burdens of those great projects,[107] and by eschewing personal publicity, he may well have been reacting defensively, attempting to preclude being held personally responsible for possible failures. In 1914, for instance, when he had instructed Allen to publicize the commission and not Hoover, he had added that "we want the Commission to become known as a responsible institution, for we may all be hung up on the barbed wire before this work is well under way."[108] And when he had asked that his name be submerged in the Food Administration, part of the reason was that the administration was "an institution, and as an institution it can withstand the shocks. An individual cannot stand all the shocks and survive."[109] This sensitivity to possible personal failure may also have been influential in keeping him from actively seeking the presidency, and it was probably one of the underlying considerations in the appeal that first an editorial and then a cabinet position had for a man of his complex personality.

In any event, Hoover relished his work at the Department of

Commerce and was quite content to remain there—at least through the summer of 1927. In January, 1923, President Harding wanted him to direct the Department of the Interior; and two years later, Coolidge asked him to become secretary of agriculture, positions that traditionally were more influential than the Commerce Department secretaryship; but Hoover, in the midst of creating a "real Department of Commerce," was convinced that he could better meet "the service needs of the whole community" by staying where he was.[110] In 1924, he asked Hubert Work, secretary of the interior, to make sure that his name was not placed in nomination for the vice-presidency. Again, he was certain that the Commerce Department afforded him an opportunity to serve in an administrative capacity of "more public importance" than the more prestigious office.[111] Nor is there any evidence to support the charge that he lusted for the presidency in either 1924 or 1928. Mark Requa, an old friend and Food Administration assistant, did function in the 1920s as an informant to Hoover on California politics and did urge him to leave the cabinet and run for the Senate or a governorship as a necessary prelude to a presidential candidacy;[112] but if Hoover ever responded to these urgings, there is no record of it at the Hoover Library or the Hoover Institution. As noted above, he was an "organization man," and so long as Coolidge wanted the presidency, he would not challenge him—no matter how strong the pressures to do so. On several occasions he repudiated efforts to promote his candidacy and disavowed news stories suggesting he aspired to the presidency. Such efforts, he kept saying, were "embarrassments," in "bad taste," and violations of his code of "honesty and decency."[113]

By 1927, though, Hoover was well aware of the strong "grass roots" political forces that had massed behind him across the country—forces that he had never acknowledged, let alone fostered. Covering the Mississippi River flood in the south for *World's Work*, Will Irwin asked his old friend, then in charge of relief operations in the area, if he was a candidate for the nomination. "I shall be the nominee, probably," Hoover had responded, "it is nearly inevitable"; but when asked what he would do should Coolidge decide to run again, he had replied, "I won't get in the way

—naturally."[114] In September, 1927, a month after Coolidge's cryptic "I do not choose to run" statement, Hoover consulted the president about his plans but received no definite answer.[115] It was at this point, and only then,[116] that he began to utilize his publicists and press connections for personal political ends. George Barr Baker, Ray Mayer, and George Akerson, all of whom had been key propagandists for the Republican National Committee in 1924,[117] were now permitted to start discreetly cultivating the press while Hoover himself consulted privately with his influential editor and columnist friends, Mark Sullivan, Frederick Wile, William Hard, William Allen White, and Frank Kent.[118]

Even so, it was not until February, 1928, that Hoover openly entered the race, and only then after he had learned from Coolidge personally that the latter was not entering the Ohio primary and had no objection to Hoover's doing so. From the time of his entrance, moreover, till the opening of the convention in June, Hoover "refused to deliver a single speech or issue a single press statement having any political connotation." So far as he was concerned "the party should make its decision on the basis of [his] public record."[119] As in 1920, he was not running for the nomination as much as making himself available. But unlike 1920, now he gave encouragement to the forces behind him, and this time they were too strong to be denied. As he had prophesied, his nomination had become "inevitable."[120]

As we have seen in this chapter, then, Herbert Hoover did employ public relations experts and did have a number of helpful acquaintances in the press during his years as secretary of commerce. But contrary to the view of his critics, this was not a result of his desire to "advertise" his own name or fulfill a burning, longstanding ambition to become president. There is no question that Hoover wanted to wield power and influence, enjoyed doing so, and used publicity to that end; but the demands of the presidency were, given his introverted nature, repugnant to him, and he did not seek the high office until he perceived that it was to be virtually handed to him. When, late in his second term as secretary of commerce, he once again gave way to the pressure of friends to make himself available for the Republican nomination, he did apparently use his press connections surreptitiously to enhance his already strong position. But this was only in the six-month period preceding the convention. In general, his heavy reliance upon public relations and the press must be seen as a means by which he could reach out to the public for support for his programs, yet remain in satisfying obscurity. An excerpt from a letter of recommendation written by Hoover in 1926 on behalf of a former subordinate in the Food Administration bears the unmistakable imprint of his own self-image: "He is a rare organizer—is not turned aside from the main goal by back eddies and by personalities; he can deal with great men and can handle the small men that seem to be attached to most movements and is always ready to work from behind the scenes—looking only for results and never to his own self glory."[121] Having now explored some of the psychological factors figuring in Hoover's behind-the-scenes style and the apparatus that he used to implement it, we must now look at the goals and results he had in mind, particularly at his philosophy and outlook, the forces shaping these, and how they complemented his style and personality.

1. Herbert Hoover to Newbold Noyes, editor of the Washington *Evening Star*, March 24, 1922, Secretary of Commerce Official File, "Associated Press," HHP, HHPL.

2. Although appreciative of Allen's services, Hoover had urged him to start "looking for something else to do" in the spring of 1919. Later in the year, he helped him purchase the Sacramento *Union*. Allen was able to keep the paper for only two years. Hoover to Ben Allen, March 18, 1919, Ben S. Allen File, Box 1, Hoover Institution on War, Peace, and Revolution; "Sacramento Union Is Sold By Allen," p. 37.

3. Baker and Rickard continued in Hoover's service as publicist and administrator of the American Relief Administration with which Hoover, though now in Washington with new duties, maintained close ties. When most of the ARA's work was completed in 1923, they remained associated with Hoover as director of public relations and administrator of the American Child Health Association of which Hoover was president from 1923 to 1935. As Hoover viewed the work of the ACHA as "a translation of our foreign [ARA] experience [with children] into American life," it was logical that he would request both men to stay on in the New York office promoting the cause of child health in America. Though their main concern at 42 Broadway was seeing to the interests of the ACHA, Baker, Rickard, and their staff also frequently operated in collaboration with Hoover's Washington office—as, for instance, in the case of the preparation, publication, and distribution of

Hoover's *American Individualism* and *Annual Report* in 1922. They also functioned in New York as unofficial Hoover press assistants, answering newspaper attacks; offering advice on speeches, press statements, and press relations; sending relevant clippings from the New York press to the Washington office; and maintaining a backlog of copies of Hoover's articles and speeches. This corpus of the "Chief's" public statements, assembled in chronological order in both the New York and Washington offices, was referred to as the "Bible" by Hoover's staff. It remains today of great assistance to researchers at the Hoover Presidential Library. SCPF, "Rickard, Edgar"; SCOF and SCPF, "Baker, George Barr," HHP, HHPL.

4. *Who's Who in America, 1928-1929* 15 (Chicago, 1928): 1022; Charles Seymour, *Letters from the Paris Peace Conference* (New Haven, Conn., 1965), p. 129.

5. *Who's Who in America, 1930-1931* 16 (Chicago, 1930): 2114.

6. George Akerson, Speech in Bronxville, New York, October 17, 1932, George E. Akerson Papers, HHPL.

7. Herbert Hoover, *The Memoirs of Herbert Hoover, 1920-1933: The Cabinet and The Presidency*, 2:43.

8. William C. Redfield was Hoover's predecessor as secretary of commerce, administering the department from 1913 to 1920 under President Wilson. Always lacking the proper appropriations with which to do an effective job—a condition of which he constantly complained in his *Annual Reports*—Redfield simply could not afford to employ publicists within the department. In his reflections upon his years in government, *With Congress and Cabinet*, he upbraids the press for its refusal to appreciate the work of cabinet officials and to treat them judiciously. Had he had the wherewithal to have done so, Redfield would have used publicists to correct misinformation in the press and to "interpret" the government "wisely" in its numerous "complex activities." He was well aware though, as Hoover himself would learn, that "organized publicity," however necessary, would bring charges that the cabinet officer was "trying to advertise" himself (William Redfield, *With Congress and Cabinet*, pp. 244-71, 280-83).

9. *Who's Who in America, 1932-1933* 17 (Chicago, 1932): 1202; Edward Eyre Hunt, *War Bread: A Personal Narrative of the War and Relief in Belgium* (New York, 1916), pp. 193-98.

10. *Who's Who in America*, 17:1202.

11. Edward Eyre Hunt, ed., *Scientific Management Since Taylor: A Collection of Authoritative Papers*, pp. xii-xiii.

12. Hunt to Ordway Tead, of the McGraw-Hill Book Co., January 23, 1922, Commerce, Colorado River Commission Records, HHP, HHPL.

13. *Who's Who in America* 15:1879; W. Sammons, vice-president of A. W. Shaw Co., to Richard Emmet, assistant to Hoover, February 11, 1922, SCOF, "Shaw, A. W.," HHP, HHPL.

14. SCOF, "Shaw, A. W., 1921-1922," HHP, HHPL.

15. *Who's Who in America* 17:818.

16. Frederick Feiker to Arch Shaw, April 20, 1921, SCOF, "Feiker, F.M., 1921-1922," HHP, HHPL.

17. Hoover to James H. McGraw, September 23, 1921, SCOF, "Feiker, F.M., 1921-1922," HHP, HHPL. McGraw and Hoover became good friends. McGraw published several special studies emerging from public inquiries inspired by Hoover. The secretary once referred to McGraw as "one of the most helpful people . . . trying to build up the Department" (Hoover to McGraw, March 21, 1923, SCOF, "Feiker, F. M., 1921-1922," HHP, HHPL).

18. Hunt to Tead, January 23, 1922, Commerce, Colorado River Commission Records, HHP, HHPL.

19. "Business Editors Will Help Hoover Solve Nation's Trade Problems," *Editor and Publisher* 53 (April 16, 1921): 11.

20. Feiker to Hoover, February 7, 1923, SCOF, "Feiker, F. M., 1923-1928," HHP, HHPL.

21. Hoover to Feiker, October 10, 1922, SCOF, "Feiker, F. M., 1921-1922," HHP, HHPL.

22. The preface to memoranda sent out from Hoover's office to all bureau and division heads in the department conveys the importance that Hoover attached to cooperation with the business editors: "A special committee from the Business Paper Editors Association called on Secretary Hoover today, and expressed a desire to obtain first-hand information as to the activities of the Department under the present Administration. The Secretary is anxious that every possible facility be rendered this committee, and to that end requests that you prepare for its use a review of the following special activities. . . ." The memoranda then specified the length and kinds of reports required of each subordinate in the department. (Harold Stokes to Bureau and Division Chiefs, September, 1924, SCOF, "Hunt, E. E., 1923-1928," HHP, HHPL). The reports were prepared in each case. Copies of them are filed in the Hoover Library under SCOF, "National Conference of Business Paper Editors, 1924," HHP, HHPL.

23. Jesse H. Neal, executive secretary of the Associated Business Papers, Inc., to Hoover, November 15, 1924, SCOF, "Neal, Jesse H.," HHP, HHPL.

24. Feiker to Hoover, January 4, 1927, SCOF, "Feiker, F. M., 1923-28," HHP, HHPL.

25. Donald Wilhelm, "Bearding the Lions," p. 21: "The Government's Own Publicity Work," p. 509.

26. "Waste Not, Want Not: An Interview with the United States Food Administrator," pp. 459-60; "Hoover and His Food Organization," pp. 283-86; "If He Were President: Herbert Hoover," pp. 170-71.

27. Wilhelm to Hoover, April 25, 1921; Hoover to William C. Mullendore, assistant to Hoover, June 12, 1922, SCOF, "Commerce—Standards, Bureau of, Wilhelm, Donald," HHP, HHPL.

28. Wilhelm to Feiker, January n.d., 1922, SCOF, "Commerce—Standards, Bureau of, Wilhelm, Donald," HHP, HHPL.

29. Wilhelm to Hoover, February 4, 1922, SCOF, "Commerce—Standards, Bureau of, Wilhelm, Donald," HHP, HHPL.

30. Wilhelm to S. W. Stratton, director of the Bureau of Standards, March 29, 1922, May 24, 1922, and November 29, 1922; Wilhelm to Wittemore, March 15, 1922; Wilhelm to Feiker, January, 1922; SCOF, "Commerce—Standards, Bureau of, Wilhelm, Donald," HHP, HHPL.

31. Pp. 407-10.

32. Hoover to Wesley L. Jones, January 26, 1922; Wilhelm to Hoover, February 4, 1922, SCOF, "Commerce—Standards, Bureau of, Wilhelm, Donald," HHP, HHPL.

33. Wilhelm, "Working with Hoover: A Close-up View of a Great and Friendly Administrator," pp. 410-16; Wilhelm to Hoover, January 20, 1922, and November 2, 1922, SCOF, "Commerce—Standards, Bureau of, Wilhelm, Donald," HHP, HHPL.

34. Paul J. Croghan to Feiker, May 28, 1921, SCOF, "Feiker, F. M., 1921-1922," HHP, HHPL.

35. In May, 1921, Feiker had recommended to Hoover the establishment of "a Bureau of Information to which all general inquiries regarding news will be directed and from which they may be redirected to the specialized division." He also had endorsed Croghan to head the department (Feiker to Hoover, May 27, 1921, SCOF, "Feiker, F. M., 1921-1922," HHP, HHPL). The press machinery subsequently set up by Hoover followed Feiker's recommendations closely.

36. Croghan to Stokes, February 10, 1926, SCOF, "Commerce, FDC, Croghan, 1926-1927." Wilhelm informed Hoover that even as of June, 1922, the number of Commerce Department publications under the new administration was already double the total issued under Redfield—and this was true even though they had been put on a sale basis (Wilhelm to Hoover, June 21, 1922, SCOF, "Commerce, Standards, Bureau of, Wilhelm, Donald," HHP, HHPL). In the fiscal year, June, 1921, to June, 1922, some 350,000 "special informational circulars" had been distributed by the department. This figure jumped steadily year by year to a point where in the single fiscal year ending June 30, 1929, some 3,626,135 circulars had been issued. Most of these works were made the subject of a press release appearing in the advance of the publication of the circular itself (F. R. Cowell, "Government Departments and the Press in the U.S.A.," pp. 220-21).

37. David Lawrence to Stokes, December 18, 1925, Secretary of Commerce Personal File, "Lawrence, David," HHP, HHPL.

38. Croghan to Herter, April 29, 1921, and January 13, 1922, SCOF, "Commerce, FDC, Croghan, 1921-1925," HHP, HHPL.

39. Croghan to Herter, January 13, 1922, SCOF, "Commerce, FDC, Croghan, 1921-1925," HHP, HHPL.

40. Leo Rosten, *The Washington Correspondents* (New York, 1937), p. 39; Herbert Corey, *The Truth About Hoover*, p. 62.

41. Hoover to Shaw, December 22, 1924; Shaw to Hoover, December 22, 1924, SCOF, "Shaw, A.W., 1923-1925"; Croghan to Stokes, December 8, 1925, SCOF, "Commerce, FDC, Croghan, 1921-1925," HHP, HHPL.

42. Croghan to Herter, December, 1921, SCOF, "Commerce, FDC, Croghan, 1921-1925," HHP, HHPL.

43. Julius Klein to Hoover, January 3, 1922, SCOF, "Press Release Service," HHP, HHPL.

44. Croghan to Klein, April 6, 1922, SCOF, "Press Release Service," HHP, HHPL.

45. Croghan to Klein, n.d., 1922, SCOF, "Publicity," HHP, HHPL.

46. The large number of clippings collected by Croghan testify to his success in reaching newspapers all across the country with his "trade opportunities" material. He penetrated not only the large metropolitan dailies but also the small dailies and weeklies of the most isolated, hinterland communities (SCOF, "Publicity," HHP, HHPL). He and Klein enjoyed celebrating their publicity successes by attaching boastful comments to the many clippings that were sent to Hoover and other members of the Department. Such unabashed comments as "if this isn't knocking 'em dead I'll sell my shirt" and "We're used to breaking into big headlines, but it ain't often that we get red ones!" convey a sense of the feverishness of the publicity activity that constantly boiled around Hoover and his department (SCOF, "Publicity," HHP, HHPL).

47. Herter to Lupton A. Wilkinson, April 2, 1921; Herter to Wilkinson, July

12, 1921; Herter to Raymond Mayer, August 3, 1921; Wilkinson to Hoover, October 13, 1922; W. C. Mullendore to Mayer, March 19, 1923, SCOF, "Wilkinson, Lupton, A.," SCPF, "Mayer, R.C.," HHP, HHPL.

48.   Hoover, Introduction to "Trade Association Activities," July 15, 1923, 319, Public Statements, HHP, HHPL.

49.   SCOF, "Bernays, Edward, L.," HHP, HHPL.

50.   John Lee Mahin to Hoover, July 5, 1922, SCOF, "Publicity," HHP, HHPL.

51.   Baker to Walter L. Brown, director of the A.R.A. London office, July 14, 1922, George Barr Baker Papers, "Lee, Ivy, L.," Box 4, Hoover Institution on War, Revolution, and Peace. On occasion, Baker would forward to his "Chief" political and economic observations prepared by members of what he called "my group of public relations men in New York"—a group including Ivy Lee with whom he lunched regularly (Baker to Hoover, June 28, 1926, George Barr Baker Papers, Box 3, Hoover Institution on War, Revolution, and Peace).

52.   Hoover to Herter, November 11, 1922, SCOF, "Commerce, Annual Report 1922, Publicity and Distribution," HHP, HHPL.

53.   Hoover to Herter, November 7, 1922, SCOF, "Commerce, Annual Report 1922, Publicity and Distribution," HHP, HHPL.

54.   Ibid.

55.   SCOF, "Annual Reports 1923, 1924, 1925, 1926," Hoover Papers.

56.   Richard Emmet to T. F. McKeon, director of department publications, November 14, 1922, SCOF, "Commerce, Annual Report 1922, Publicity and Distribution," HHP, HHPL.

57.   Croghan to Emmet, November, 1923, SCOF, "Annual Report, 1923," HHP, HHPL.

58.   In November, 1922, Hoover instructed one of his departmental assistants, William Mullendore, who had been on the legal staff of the Food Administration and had prepared the official history of that organization, to send a statement containing the sentiments expressed above to *System* magazine (Mullendore to Arch Shaw, November 7, 1922, SCOF, "Shaw, A.W., 1921-1922," HHP, HHPL).

59.   As noted in the preceding chapter, *Bookman, Collier's, Dun's Review, Independent, Ladies' Home Journal, Leslie's Weekly, Life, Literary Digest, Outlook, Town Topics,* and *World's Work* all "gave generous space" to the CRB and "donated advertising for contributions." Edward Bok of the *Ladies' Home Journal* and R. J. Cuddihy of the *Literary Digest* undertook special private campaigns for funds that were then turned over to the CRB (Gay and Fisher, *Public Relations of the Commission for Relief in Belgium,* 2:245-46). Magazine and newspaper space was also liberally given the Food Administration for its propaganda (Mullendore, *The History of the United States Food Administration, 1917-1919,* pp. 83-86, 88).

60.   Henry F. May has noted the recurrence of the phrase "practical idealism" in American magazines and newspapers in the decade before World War I. Popularly regarded as a uniquely American creed, practical idealism, of which the Social Gospel was one important manifestation, assumed that ideals were inextricably linked to material achievement and should be kept within the range of actual realization (*The End of American Innocence,* pp. 9-19). Hoover's CRB, Food Administration, and postwar relief work became for many Amercians tangible expressions of the nation's exemplary code of practical idealism. Hoover's "matter-of-fact idealism"—which became especially attractive when contrasted with the failure of Wilson's "abstract idealism" at Versailles—was thus the quality that his close friends and a whole host of admirers in the press singled out for praise and publicity. See

for example: Vernon Kellogg, "Herbert Hoover as Individual and Type," pp. 384-85; Kellogg, "Washington Five and Eight O'Clocks," pp. 460-61; Kellogg, *Herbert Hoover: The Man and His Work*, p. 125; Will Irwin, "Hoover As an Executive," p. 5; French Strother, "Herbert Hoover: Representative American and Practical Idealist," pp. 578-85; Julius Barnes, "Herbert Hoover: Some Reasons for His Reputation," pp. 642-44. In one of many public tributes to Hoover, a Dartmouth College Commencement official, conferring an honorary degree upon him in June, 1920, eulogized him as the "eloquent spokesman of a great nation's better self and an exponent to stricken peoples of its practical idealism" (New York *Evening Post*, June 23, 1920).

61. [George Horace Lorimer], "Demosthenes and Democracy," p. 28.

62. Will Irwin to Hoover, December n.d., 1919, and February 7, 1920, Pre-Commerce Correspondence, Hoover Papers; Irwin, "Hoover as an Executive," pp. 192-95.

63. Herbert Hoover, "Some Notes on Agricultural Adjustment," *Saturday Evening Post* 192 (April 10, 1920): 3-4; "Announcement," *Saturday Evening Post* 193 (November 20, 1920): 25.

64. Norman Hapgood to Hoover, April n.d., 1920, Pre-Commerce Correspondence, HHP, HHPL; "Elect Hoover, Hapgood Urges," Philadelphia *Ledger*, April 13, 1920.

65. Hartford Powel to Hoover, November 28, 1921, SCOF, "Collier's Weekly," HHP, HHPL. On April 9, 1921, Powel had run an editorial, effusive in its praise of Hoover, in order "to get the American public, or a million members of it, at any rate, thinking seriously about the Department of Commerce" (Powel to Herter, March 22, 1921, SCOF, "Collier's Weekly," HHP, HHPL).

66. SCPF, "Marcosson, Isaac," HHP, HHPL.

67. Marcosson to Hoover, January 22, 1926, SCPF, "Marcosson, Isaac," HHP, HHPL. A reviewer of *Caravans of Commerce* was quick to observe that Marcosson had been a "good press agent." He complained that *"Caravans of Commerce* as a title is wrong; the book should have been called *Hoover's Sagacity in the Department of Commerce*. It is a lengthy hymn on the achievements of the Secretary of that department" (Adonis Syvil, "Marcosson's New Book on Herbert Hoover Is Good Press Agenting," Houston *Post*, November 7, 1926, SCPF, "Marcosson, Isaac," HHP, HHPL).

68. Hoover to George H. Lorimer, May 26, 1923, SCPF, "Saturday Evening Post," HHP, HHPL.

69. Hoover to Lorimer, June 1, 1923, SCOF, "Lorimer, George H.," HHP, HHPL.

70. Samuel Blythe, "A Calm View of a Calm Man," p. 73. Interestingly enough it was this article that Mrs. Harding was reading to the president when he died in his San Francisco hotel suite (E. W. Starling, *Starling of the White House*, p. 200; Mark Sullivan, *Our Times: The Twenties*, 6:250.

71. Hoover to Lorimer, June 17, 1927, SCPF, "Saturday Evening Post," HHP, HHPL.

72. Hoover to Lorimer, July 7, 1927, SCPF, "Saturday Evening Post," HHP, HHPL.

73. William Allen White has recorded his first impression of Hoover upon hearing him deliver a short talk on behalf of the CRB before a small group of people in New York in 1915: "We found Herbert Hoover a most intelligent person who smiled naively with a certain vinegary integrity, a person with a most delicious sense of

humor. . . . That whole group [of "twelve to fifteen people"] . . . was mesmerized by the strange low voltage of his magnetism. Sallie [White's wife] and I felt and we had met a Person—a Person of some dignity and power" (William Allen White, *The Autobiography of William Allen White*, p. 515). Hamilton Holt, who first met Hoover in Paris early in 1919, recalled: "In response to a question in regard to the world situation he [Hoover] launched out upon a forty-minute monologue, the like of which I have never heard from any mortal man before or since. Although he spoke with a range and sweep that included armies, nations, and even continents as though they were pawns in a game, his knowledge was fortified by fact and details. Never have I been more enthralled by charm of the spoken word or by sheer brilliancy of thought, analysis, and exposition. I was in the presence of a master" (Hamilton Holt, "When Mr. Hoover Talks," p. 589). Paul Y. Anderson, who became one of Hoover's most acerbic press critics during his presidency, reported after an interview with Hoover in 1925: "To say that Secretary Hoover talked interestingly is superfluous. Hoover is always interesting. When Presidents want a difficult job done thoroughly, Hoover usually gets the call, especially if the job requires actual technical knowledge. . . . When Washington correspondents cannot get needed information elsewhere, they invariably try Hoover, regardless of whether it comes under his department. He generally has it or knows where it can be obtained. The scope of his interests and the range of his information is astonishing" (Paul Y. Anderson, "Economic Situation in Nation Best in Our History Says Hoover," *St. Louis Post-Dispatch*, October 19, 1925, 514, Public Statements, HHP, HHPL). In 1926, James O'Donnell Bennett gave a vivid account of Hoover's effectiveness in relating to the press after presenting a report before a congressional committee: "A dozen newspaper correspondents who have sat, listening and note taking, at a side table for two hours, crowd around him to ask him to verify amazing facts and enormous figures in the talk he just has finished. He verifies . . . and you feel his intense desire that the facts be accurately and clearly understood. . . . Next morning, newspapers a thousand miles distant print a column or more of what Hoover said to the Committee. Next day come the editorials. Thus Hoover—sedate, laconic, undramatic, berating nobody, asserting nothing that his laboriously gathered facts and figures will not sustain—draws a picture that everybody understands. And he again has walked away with the day's publicity in the publicity center of the Republic. . . . And that is why he is the despair and wonder of the fame-famished in Washington" (James O'Donnell Bennett, "Marching with Hoover to the Sea," *Liberty*, May 22, 1926, p. 584, Public Statements, HHP, HHPL).

74.   SCOF, "Mark Sullivan"; SCOF, "Senate, Arthur Capper"; SCOF and SCPF, "William Allen White"; SCOF, "Richard Oulahan"; SCPF, "Frederick W. Wile"; SCOF and SCPF, "William Hard"; SCOF and SCPF, "David Lawrence"; SCOF and SCPF, "Gertrude B. Lane"; SCPF, "Ida Tarbell"; SCOF, "Edward G. Lowry," HHP, HHPL.

75.   James L. McCamy, *Government Publicity: Its Practice in Federal Administration*, p. 12; F. R. Cowell, "Government Departments and the Press in the U.S.A." pp. 216, 220.

76.   Alfred W. McCann complained in the October, 1917, *Forum* that "an efficient department store manager or train dispatcher could have done the C.R.B. job as well as Hoover"—and "with a press agent as skillful as the metallurgist's, they would have become equally famous." McCann was convinced that "the preparation of the American mind by Hoover, to accept Hoover was undertaken with adroit persistence" (Alfred W. McCann, "The Hoover Food-Control Failure," pp. 382-83). Clinton W. Gilbert, who was certain Hoover had presidential ambitions, was of the opinion that Hoover's "one great gift [was] his extraordinary talent for

publicity." His sudden fame during the war had resulted from "his own instinct for publicity, his sense of what interests the people, his assiduous cultivation of editors and reporters." He had "magazine and newspaper contacts only exceeded by those of Theodore Roosevelt in his time, and a sense of the power of publicity only exceeded by Roosevelt" ([Clinton W. Gilbert], *The Mirrors of Washington*, pp. 120-21).

77. Victoria Allen, "The Outside Man," 1:37, Ben Allen Papers, HHPL. Will Irwin, recalling his days in the commission's New York office, has written: "Newspapers and magazines, scenting a story, began appealing for 'personality stuff' on Hoover. He would stand for nothing of the sort. 'Play up the need in Belgium: keep me out of it,' he cabled" (Irwin, *Herbert Hoover: A Reminiscent Biography*, pp. 175-76).

78. Gay and Fisher, *Public Relations of the Commission for Relief in Belgium*, 1:4-5, 9; Irwin, *Herbert Hoover*, p. 175.

79. Allen, "The Outside Man," 1:37.

80. Hoover, "Bind the Wounds of France," 1-C, Public Statements, HHP, HHPL.

81. Hoover, "Conserving the Food Supply," 3-F, Public Statements, HHP, HHPL.

82. Edward Bok to Hoover, October 19, 1917, Pre-Commerce Correspondence, HHP, HHPL.

83. Food Administration Files, "Press Releases," HHP, HHPL.

84. *Who's Hoover?*, pp. 155-56.

85. Hoover to Mason Peters (editor of the *Journal of Commerce*), December 9, 1921, SCOF, "Press Release Service," HHP, HHPL.

86. Stokes to Croghan, June n.d., 1925, SCOF, "Commerce, FDC, Croghan, 1921-1925," HHP, HHPL.

87. John Marrinan (assistant to Hoover) to Croghan, March 20, 1926, SCOF, "Commerce, FDC, Croghan, 1926-1927," HHP, HHPL. Hoover once wrote his good friend Frederick Wile asking that he amend some statements made in praise of him in the Washington *Star*. He feared that Wile's article would "cause an overestimation of [his] services" unless it was corrected (Hoover to Wile, January 29, 1925, SCPF, "Wile, Frederick W.," HHP, HHPL).

88. Hoover's personal copy of William Hard's biography of him was also dedicated "to the victim" (Ray T. Tucker, "Is Hoover Human?," p. 515).

89. Irwin to Hoover, February 7, 1920, Pre-Commerce Correspondence, HHP, HHPL.

90. "Working with Hoover," 413.

91. Ibid., p. 414.

92. Alfred P. Dennis, "Humanizing the Department of Commerce," p. 8.

93. Hugh Gibson, "Herbert Clark Hoover," p. 517.

94. Hoover to Charles T. Neal, September 24, 1919, Pre-Commerce Correspondence, HHP, HHPL.

95. Hoover to Harry C. Riddle, October 3, 1919, Pre-Commerce Correspondence, HHP, HHPL. This was a rather stock reply for Hoover at this time. When Ray Stannard Baker sent Hoover a newspaper clipping in which he had expressed the hope that "the administrator" would seek the presidency, Hoover had written back: "Everybody likes words of commendation more especially from people whom one esteems as highly as I do yourself. On the other hand, I am convinced that you

are somewhat on the wrong track, for I have a notion that what this country needs is a few private citizens, as well as aspirants for public office" (Hoover to Baker, October 6, 1919, Pre-Commerce Correspondence, HHP, HHPL).

96.   Hoover to William A. Glascow, April 12, 1919, Pre-Commerce Correspondence, HHP, HHPL. Hoover's sensitivity to "political mud" was so great that even occasional harebrained attacks on his Food Administration—attacks overwhelmed by the general acclaim accorded him—once caused him to complain that he had "drunk of the bitterness of public life to such a depth that no inducement short of national danger would ever bring [him] again into public life" (Hoover to Mark L. Requa, February 21, 1919, George Barr Baker Papers, Box 6, Hoover Institution on War, Revolution, and Peace).

97.   Caspar W. Hodgson to Hoover, September 24, 1919; Hoover to Hodgson, September 29, 1919, Pre-Commerce Correspondence, HHP, HHPL.

98.   Hoover to Hodgson, February 12, 1920, Pre-Commerce Correspondence, HHP, HHPL. Hoover did issue a press release assuring the American public that he was not a British citizen as a Hearst paper had alleged. He began the statement, which was released February 5, 1920, by again insisting: "I am not seeking the Presidency; I know something of what the burdens of that office are. I am not a candidate. I have no organization. No one is authorized to speak for me politically."

99.   Hoover to Ralph Arnold, March 8, 1920, 50, Public Statements, HHP, HHPL.

100.   Hoover to Warren Gregory, March 30, 1920, Pre-Commerce Correspondence, HHP, HHPL.

101.   Statement re Nomination, April 3, 1920, 56, Public Statements, HHP, HHPL.

102.   Quoted by unidentified correspondent to Hugh Gibson, March 6, 1920, Ray Lyman Wilbur Papers, "Political—1920," Hoover Institution on War, Revolution, and Peace; Hoover, *Memoirs*, 2:35; White, *Autobiography*, pp. 586-88.

103.   Robert K. Murray, "President Harding and His Cabinet," *Ohio History* 75 (Spring-Summer, 1966):113-14.

104.   Quoted in Barry D. Karl, "Presidential Planning and Social Science Research," *Perspectives in American History* 3 (1969):353.

105.   Hoover to Glascow, April 12, 1919, Pre-Commerce Correspondence, HHP, HHPL.

106.   In the period 1919-20, Hoover purchased shares in the Sacramento *Union* and the Washington *Herald*. In 1919, he actually performed editorial work for the *Herald*, meeting frequently with the paper's manager and reporters to discuss the *Herald's* affairs (Willis J. Abbot, *Watching the World Go By*, p. 312). In these same years, Hoover was interested in buying into the New York *Herald* and the Baltimore *Sun*. His plans concerning these latter two papers, however, never materialized (Gerald W. Johnson, Frank Kent, H. L. Mencken, and Hamilton Owens, *The Sunpapers of Baltimore* [New York, 1937], p. 313; George Britt, *Forty Years—Forty Millions: The Career of Frank A. Munsey*, p. 256). An attempt to purchase another newspaper, the San Francisco *Chronicle*, which Hoover made through one of his publicity aides, George Barr Baker, was also unsuccessful at this time (George Barr Baker to Roy M. Pike, December 1, 1919; Baker to Hoover, December n.d., 1919, Boxes 5 and 3, George Barr Baker Papers, Hoover Institution on War, Revolution, and Peace).

107.   In examining Hoover's pre-1914 career in the first and second chapters, we encountered a strange duality in his personality: an aggressive desire to move

men and events that was countered by a markedly "retiring" aspect in his nature. Although the aggressive element of his make-up spurred him to seek entry into public life, the "retiring" side made actually doing so very difficult for him. This same ambivalence remained with Hoover as he contemplated his work with the CRB and the Food Administration. Will Irwin well remembered Hoover's agonizing over whether or not to direct the CRB: "He didn't know [whether to accept] for three tormented days, during which the [American] Embassy had him under steady pressure. He talked little when at home. My room at Red House was under his, and every night I woke to hear the steady, distant beat of his footsteps. As is his habit, when in perplexity or deep thought, he was walking the floor—and doubtless jingling the coins or keys in his pocket" (Irwin, *The Making of a Reporter*, p. 252). And Edward Bok recalled Hoover musing, shortly after becoming food administrator, "I don't know why I am in this thing." When Bok asked how he had got into it, Hoover had replied, "I don't know, sort of forced into it" (Edward Bok, *Twice Thirty* p. 296).

108. Allen, "The Outside Man," 1:147.

109. Hoover, "Conserving the Food Supply," 3-F, Public Statements, HHP, HHPL.

110. Refusal of Secretaryship of Department of Interior, January 6, 1923, 278, Public Statements, HHP, HHPL; Refusal of Secretaryship of Department of Agriculture, January 16, 1925, 436, Public Statements, HHP, HHPL.

111. Hoover to Hubert B. Work, June 5, 1924, SCPF, HHP, HHPL.

112. SCPF, "Mark Requa," HHP, HHPL.

113. In the spring of 1923, Hoover wrote to a would-be supporter: "I am told that at a recent Stanford meeting someone made a statement looking to support for me as a presidential candidate next election. This sort of thing is of the most embarrassing character. Obviously, every sense of honesty and decency requires that nothing of this kind should be done by myself or my friends" (Hoover to William Snow, May 1, 1923, SCPF, HHP, HHPL). In 1925, he wrote to a correspondent of the Baltimore *Sun* protesting an article entitled, "Boom for Hoover in 1928." He complained that "the writer of the story [had] taken up a usual fulsome after-dinner introduction speech directed at myself, which was neither intended nor in any way bears the interpretation given the article published by the *Sun*. Neither the speaker nor the audience made any such assumption for none of them were possessed of such bad taste" (Hoover to Fred Essary, April 27, 1925, SCPF, HHP, HHPL). Donald Wilhelm, in a clumsy attempt to regain employment as a publicist in the department, once offered to organize a secret publicity campaign "smearing" Hoover's political adversaries within the Republican party, Hiram Johnson and Gifford Pinchot. Hoover replied to this suggestion briefly and cuttingly: "I have your letter of January 19th. I have always taken the attitude that I will not mix in this sort of thing. If it is necessary as a part of public service, then I shall go out of public service" (Hoover to Wilhelm, January 22, 1924, SCPF, HHP, HHPL).

114. Irwin, *The Making of a Reporter*, p. 409.

115. Hoover, *Memoirs*, 2:190.

116. George Akerson has commented that it was only after Coolidge had removed himself from contention that Hoover "permitted any of us to make a move looking to his nomination at the subsequent Republican Convention" (Akerson, Speech in Bronxville, New York, October 17, 1932, George E. Akerson Papers, HHPL). Lewis L. Strauss, whose own career began as a Hoover secretary during the years 1917-19 and who always maintained close ties with his "Chief," has written in his autobiography: "Mr. Hoover had told us in no uncertain terms that he

was not a candidate and would not consider the subject until Mr. Coolidge had made his own intentions plain" (Lewis L. Strauss, *Men and Decisions*, p. 54).

117.   George Barr Baker Papers, "Coolidge, Calvin," Hoover Institution on War, Revolution, and Peace.

118.   Bradley Nash, who served on Hoover's secretarial staff from 1927 to 1929, has recently recalled that he arrived at his job in September, 1927, right at the time when Hoover was beginning to meet in his office with "the publishers, feature writers, and analysts" mentioned above. Nash agreed with Raymond Henle's comment that, in the fall and winter of 1927, Hoover was "preparing for the nomination" by "seeing many people of influence" (Bradley Nash interviewed by Raymond Henle, director, Herbert Hoover Oral History Program, July 31, 1968, HHPL).

119.   Hoover, *Memoirs*, 2:191.

120.   Christian Herter, Hoover's former press secretary, observed shortly after the convention: "The nomination of Herbert Hoover as the Republican standard bearer did not take place at Kansas City: it was merely ratified there. Months, even years before, a small army of men and women dotted all over the United States formed a group of missionaries whose work had been accomplished long before June 12. These were the men and women who had served with Mr. Hoover during the past in one or more of his many gigantic enterprises" (Christian Herter, "Looking Back on Kansas City," p. 614).

121.   Hoover to Mrs. George T. Gerlinger, member of the Board of Regents of the University of Oregon, February 13, 1926, SCPF, "Short, William H.," HHP, HHPL.

5 Educating the Masses

IN THE PRECEDING CHAPTERS, Herbert Hoover's extraordinary public relations machinery, personnel, and press contacts have been explained in terms of his personality and the idiosyncratic, behind-the-scenes style of administration that grew out of it. In the present chapter, the analysis of his public relations style will be extended by placing it in the context of his progressive social outlook and political philosophy. Old myths about his social and political thought die hard,[1] yet, in outlook and philosophy, and in the publicity strategy that these entailed, it becomes clear that he belongs to the progressive political tradition of early twentieth-century America. Far from expounding Sumnerian laissez-faire principles and far from embodying the ascendancy of self-interested business forces, as he has so frequently been represented,[2] he emerges, particularly from his hitherto largely neglected public statements from 1917 to 1921, as one of the foremost public figures bearing the banners of prewar progressivism into the 1920s.

I

"One looming shadow of this war is its drift toward social disruption. . . ." So spoke Hoover in September, 1917, as he eyed the Russian government and social structure in the process of disintegration.[3] From 1917 through his presidency, the threat of social disruption would loom large in his social outlook. An intelligent student of societies the world over and a man with great personal experience in, and knowledge of, international economics and diplomacy, Hoover had been uniquely prepared and, from his vantage point as chairman of the CRB, uniquely positioned to comprehend the catastrophic consequences of World War I for all of Western civilization.[4] What he would come to view as the "happiest period of all humanity in the Western World in ten centuries"—the twenty-five years preceding the conflict[5]—had come to an abrupt end. An international order, which the diffusion of economic security, scientific research, and public education seemed to be progressively stabilizing, had been shattered,[6] resulting in the complete breakdown of international commerce, the economic deprivation of millions of people, and the inflammation of class conflicts and nationalistic hatreds. All of this had impressed Hoover, vividly and lastingly, with the fragility of the world order as well as the social fabric of all the industrialized countries of the West, including the United States. Consequently, a concern for the stability of international society and, after 1919, especially for that of the American social order became the dominant feature of his social outlook and the spur behind all his public policies from 1920 to 1932.

Even before the Armistice, Hoover realized that the Wilsonian aim of subverting the "autocracies in Europe and . . . establish[ing] . . . government by the people" was only a "part of the great burden" of the United States in establishing a secure world order. The greatest problem lay in "nursing Europe back to industry and self support" through the distribution of food and medical supplies collected in America. Only this would "prevent Europe's immolation in a conflagration of anarchy such as Russia is plunged in today."[7] Thus, when the fighting ceased, Hoover, as we have seen, saw to it that his Food Administration machinery, which had operated to help the Allies win the war, was kept intact and functioning. It could now be used "to provision the allies and the liberated nations of Europe [including Germany] which face not hunger alone but the collapse of all that holds civilization together."[8] And in his public statements, designed to raise funds for the American Relief Administration, he kept hammering away at this theme. Famine was the "mother of anarchy," and unless "stability of government was obtained in the enemy states, there would be nobody to pay reparations to France and Belgium";[9] only if the United States finished its job of provisioning Europe could it banish "the spectre of Bolshevism," which was attempting "to lure the distressed peoples into such hopeless misery and anarchy as now afflicts Russia";[10] if the United States valued "its own safety," the "social organization of the world," and the "preservation of civilization itself," it must act against "this cancer in the world's vitals" —famine, anarchy, and Bolshevism;[11] looking at the international situation "from the most selfish point of view of our own future interests," there could be no peace and recuperation of trade if the United States permitted "the creation of another cesspool like Russia."[12] Similarly, Hoover's intense concern for a secure social and economic world order made him a strong advocate of American participation in the League of Nations. For unless the European nations, old and new, had a "generation of actual national life in peace to develop free education and skill in government," unless they "had a guiding hand and referee in their quarrels, a court of appeal for their wrongs," all Europe would "go back to chaos." Without peace and without economic security, the "safety of European civilization" would remain "hanging by a slender thread."[13]

During these same years (1917-20), Hoover was also concerned with internal threats to the American social order. As food administrator, he had been all too aware that the wartime disruption of the international price mechanism could be exploited to great personal advantage by unscrupulous speculators in the American grain and livestock markets. The resulting higher food prices, he feared, would catch American labor in a price-wage scissors, which, in time, would lead to social unrest and disrupt the war mobilization effort. There would be a growth of "class feeling formed by the unusual privations of the war,"[14] resulting in "strikes, disorder, riots, and the defeat of our national efficiency."[15] Uncontrolled speculation and profiteering, demonstrating the "failure of commerce to serve the public interest," might make "the condition of the industrial classes so intolerable as to steam the hotbed of revolution," just as a similar "failure of the government and the commercial classes to meet their public duty"[16] in Russia had produced revolution there. He therefore established price controls on food commodities at the wholesale level and, in his Food Administration propaganda, urged frugality in the purchase and consumption of food, not only to conserve it, but also to restrain the tendency toward rising food prices.[17]

When Hoover returned from his overseas supervision of the European relief program in September, 1919, his concern for American social and economic stability was heightened by the postwar condition of the country. As he recalls in his *Memoirs*:

> It was apparent that from war, inflation, overexpanded agriculture, great national debt, delayed housing and postponed modernization of industry, demoralization of our foreign trade, high taxes, and swollen bureaucracy, we were faced with the need for reconstruction at home. . . . We were neglecting the primary obligations of health and education of our children over large backward areas. Most of our employers were concertedly fighting the legitimate development of trade unions, and thereby stimulating the emergence of radical leaders and, at the same time, class cleavage. The twelve-hour day and eighty-four-hour week were still extant in many industries.[18]

Though speechmaking was "not a treasured part of [his] life" and though he realized he was "no spellbinder," Hoover nevertheless felt compelled to speak out on the issues and did so in forty-six public addresses delivered between October, 1919, and March, 1921,[19]—addresses often reaching a national audience through the publicity efforts of George Barr Baker and Edgar Rickard out of the ARA office.[20] In this same period, he also gave out thirty-one press statements, wrote twenty-eight magazine articles, and made four extensive reports—all bearing on his concern for postwar reconstruction and development.[21] In these many statements, Hoover expressed the fear that unless steps were taken to solve the problems stemming from labor-management antagonisms, wasteful industrial practices, "vicious speculation," the lack of housing, and inadequate child health facilities, "the community [would be] torn to pieces by impossible class conflicts."[22] And to prevent such a catastrophe, he turned naturally to his fellow engineers and called upon them to study and "give voice to the critical matters of national policy" so essential to the welfare of the nation.[23] Given the complexity, fragility, and needs of American society, he had come to feel, only the experience, training, and empirical attitude of the engineer, scientist, and businessman could solve the social and economic problems.[24] He would shortly add the economist to this group, and his elitism, his belief in the indispensability of the expert in the management of government and society, would become explicit.[25]

In addition to enumerating the problems unsettling American society and sketching solutions for them, Hoover's statements of the immediate postwar period also attempted to define an American political and social philosophy within which corrective policies could be carried out. They contained, in other words, most of the elements of his later book, *American Individualism*, which he regarded as a "definition [of] the actual permanent and persistent motivation of our civilization."[26] By the autumn of 1919, he was already proclaiming his "greater appreciation of the enormous distance that we of America have grown away from Europe in the century and a half of our national existence."[27] Europe, for him, had become "a boiling social and economic caldron," casting off "miasmic infections"[28] that threatened the health and purity of the American social philosophy—a philosophy that "the American people [had] been steadily developing for generations," one that "had stood this period of test in the fire of common sense,"[29] and one that "in substance" was built on the idea of "equality of opportunity—an equal chance—to every citizen. . . ." "Its stimulus," he declared in statement after statement, "is competition. Its safeguard is education. Its greatest mentor is free speech and voluntary organization for the public good."[30] Through America's "own national institutions,"[31] he argued, through the school, the church, local and state government, through associations, and through charitable organizations like the Red Cross, Community Chest, YMCA, and settlement house, all institutions that he had worked closely with and grown to admire greatly, it was possible to resolve the great social problems of the day without scrapping such "national instincts" as individual initiative, equal opportunity, and local responsibility, and without resorting to the "dangers of centralized and federally imposed control."[32]

As the above sentence indicates, Hoover's social and political philosophy found no place for a dynamic national government. His fear of the federal government's becoming centralized in an all-powerful national bureaucracy was as old as his Food Administration days and something he carried with him to his grave. Although acutely aware of the interdependence and fragility of modern American society, of "a great but delicate cobweb in which each part must maintain its precise relation to every other part,"[33] he always maintained that increased federal power was not the way to hold the system together, that, on the contrary, the growth of a national bureaucracy would only make the tasks more difficult. By undermining individual initiative and local responsibility, it would "destroy the productivity of the people and diminish the standards of living," just as the "radical bureaucracy" of Russia and the "autocratic" one of Germany had done in those countries.[34] Repeatedly in his speeches of the 1919-20 period, he warned his audiences of the "imported social diseases"—socialism and Bolshevism—which "in these days of intimate communication" were "rapid in their penetration and infection,"[35] and which, unless militantly resisted by the "constant constructive animation of our own ideals,"[36] might endanger the American social system by fostering the weakening of "initiative in our people and the political domination that can grow from governmental operation."[37] As food administrator, he had noted on several occasions that the "difference between democracy and autocracy is a question of whether people can be organized from the bottom up or from the top down."[38] During the war, he noted with some pride, he had been successful in achieving the former, thereby avoiding "Prussianizing" the American people through a federally imposed rationing system.[39] And later, as secretary of commerce and as president, he would remain convinced that organization from the "bottom up" was the only viable manner of administering to the needs of American society. Those who disagreed with him and argued for increased federal regulation or for governmental ownership and operation of industry were "homegrown Bolsheviks."

II

Hoover's widely discredited presidency, the great popular and scholarly enthusiasm for the New Deal that followed, and perhaps his militant ideological anticommunism have obscured for most historians the fact that he was a "progressive" politically and in his social outlook. The inaccessibility, until recently, of primary sources pertaining to his pre-presidential career has also helped to perpetuate the distorted view of him as a conservative figure from the business world whose career in government was motivated primarily by a desire to promote the interests of big business and industry.[40] Even now, since little can be known about his pre-1914 career, it is difficult to establish fully his links with the reform currents that moved through American society in the years 1901 through 1916. But the fact is clear that these links did exist, even though he was outside the country much of the time. The ethic of disinterested "public service," of being "above" any class or special interest and working for the commonwealth, was characteristic not only of the developing profession of engineering but also of the progressive mood; and, as we have seen, Hoover fully subscribed to it and was moved by it to contemplate entry into "public service."[41] Evidently, he was also keeping in touch with progressive issues and personalities in these years. In 1912 he contributed a thousand dollars to Theodore Roosevelt's campaign fund,[42] and once he began his public career, many of his closest relationships were with members of the progressive camp. Both James D. Phelan and Franklin K. Lane, who had been active progressives in California and had then moved on to Washington,[43] were good friends of Hoover and were able to assist him considerably when he came to Washington in 1917 and undertook the organization of the Food Administration.[44] Such close friends as Will Irwin, George Barr Baker, and Lawrence Richey were also intimately connected with the prewar reform movement. Irwin, who had kept in touch with Hoover ever since their Stanford University days, was well-known and respected for his reform-minded journalism.[45] Baker, a Hoover aide from the CRB days through the presidency, had been an associate editor of *Everybody's Magazine* from 1907 to

1910—the period of *Everybody's* most intense interest in exposure journalism.[46] And in these same years, Richey, who became Hoover's "confidential assistant" during the Food Administration period and remained with him in such a capacity through his presidency, had used his detective experience and training as an investigator for *Everybody's*. In this work, he had ferreted out information used by reformers C. P. Connolly and Judge Ben B. Lindsey in their articles for the magazine.[47]

In March, 1920, shortly before he reluctantly made himself available for the Republican presidential nomination, Hoover described his political allegiances as "Progressive Republican before the war," "non-partisan during the war service," and "independent progressive in the issues before us today."[48] This assessment is borne out by his speeches and articles of the 1917-20 period. Repeatedly, for example, he developed the progressive theme of stewardship and responsibility for the underprivileged in society. "The justification of any rich man in the community," he maintained, "is his trusteeship to the community for his wealth. . . . The ownership of his wealth carries serious dangers . . . and behooves its trustees to take account of its responsibilities." Or similarly, he argued that the advance of civilization depended upon "the tempering of the struggle for existence by the cure of the helpless. The survival of the strong, the development of the individual, must be tempered, or else we return two thousand years in our civilization."[49]

The prewar progressives had also viewed themselves as mediating between conflicting social ideologies and classes in the interest of the public good,[50] a posture that Hoover now adopted. He saw himself as representing "progressive democracy," which sought progress through the maintenance of "individual initiative" and "equal opportunity," but was being challenged from both the right and the left. On the right, it was threatened by "reaction," which sought, "at its best, to maintain things as they are," and, "at its worst, to dominate by a narrow class that expects the great mass of people to serve their special interest." On the left, it was challenged by "radicalism embracing various degrees of socialism," which had "no patience with the gradual upbuilding of progress," and sought bureaucratic domination of society in government ownership and operation of public utilities.[51] In the past, this progressive democracy had produced the regulatory legislation that marked a definite "abandonment of the unrestricted capitalism of Adam Smith"[52] and stood as "a monument to our attempt to limit economic domination, to give a square deal." And now, by calling for cooperation from "all our economic groups," it was providing a "new economic system based neither on the capitalism of Adam Smith nor upon the socialism of Karl Marx,"[53] one that in reality offered a "third alternative that preserved individual initiative and stimulated it through protection from domination" by either the right or the left.[54]

As an "independent progressive," Hoover also recognized labor's right to unionize and bargain collectively through representatives of its own choosing. This was a matter both of economic justice and of insuring economic stability, since "extremists on both sides" threatened the disruption and domination of society. To achieve justice, he would recognize "the human right to consolidate the worker in the proper balanced position . . . against the consolidation of capital."[55] And to achieve stability, he would work to discover the areas of "common interest" between labor and management and to find measures by which through cooperation the field of common interest could be organized [and] the area of conflict eliminated." The vast majority of workers and union leaders, he felt, were "individualistic" in their social outlook,[56] and hence by recognizing the American Federation of Labor and its legitimate demands for a more equitable distribution of wealth, American management and society in general would actually erect a major "bulwark against socialism."[57]

In addition to his liberal attitudes toward industrial relations, Hoover was clearly connected to the prewar progressives through his interest in a variety of other social and economic issues. He spoke often, for instance, of the need to protect the interests of the "unorganized public" against "vicious speculators," and the need to maintain "the present inheritance, income, and excess profits taxes" in order to "control corporations" and prevent the "unrestricted accumulation of wealth" in the hands of "a narrow group of holders." As a legacy of his Belgian and postwar relief work, he became vitally interested in child health and welfare and established ties with social workers such as Homer Folks. In speeches before charitable societies and statements in *Better Times*, a "social betterment" publication, he addressed himself to problems related to urbanization and immigration. And underlying all these issues was his great concern for the maintenance of traditional American institutions and values threatened by rapid social change.[58]

Not surprisingly, many of the celebrated prewar progressive intellectuals pushed for his nomination for president in 1920. Louis Brandeis, for instance, well known as the "people's lawyer" of the progressive era, wrote Norman Hapgood that he was "100 per cent for" Hoover. "High public spirit, extraordinary intelligence, knowledge, sympathy, youth, and a rare perception of ability and power of inspiring loyalty," he believed, "would do wonderful things in the Presidency." Harvard economist and reformer Frank W. Taussig wrote Hoover that he would vote for him "on any ticket whatever, republican, democratic, new faith, socialistic, or Bolshevik." He could scarcely express "how complete [his] faith and how great [his] admiration" was for him. Edward A. Ross, sociologist and author of the influential progressive social critique *Sin and Society* (1907) informed Hoover that he was "getting in on the ground floor of the movement in Wisconsin which is for you for President." A letter of his to the *Wisconsin State Journal*, Ross regarded as the "opening gun of the . . . movement on your behalf."[59] In this same period and shortly thereafter, other progressive intellectuals also addressed to Hoover their expressions of admiration and respect.[60]

As a progressive, then, Hoover was intensely concerned with a multitude of problems jeopardizing the stability and well-being of postwar America. Labor unrest, industrial inefficiency, the wildly fluctuating business cycle, the stagnation of American foreign trade, inadequate housing and child health facilities, the menace of alien ideologies—all of these threatened the American social order, required immediate attention, and could not be adequately or safely handled without the expertise of a skilled elite, made up particularly of the engineer, the scientist, the economist, and the businessman. Yet, though Hoover's recognition of this made him a social engineering elitist, he was also a passionate democrat, convinced that American society must be run from the "bottom up." Unlike some "advanced" progressives, he felt that augmented federal powers would only undermine the individual initiative and responsibility that constituted the essence of democracy as well as the mainspring of progress. The big question was how best to bridge the gap between the expert and the citizen. How could one achieve stability in a complex industrial society without sacrificing the democratic right and obligation of participation by all individuals in that society? How could he preserve and respect local institutions while using them in the solution of pressing national problems? For Hoover, when he became secretary of commerce, the answer would be publicity and public relations. Just as these had been used in the CRB and Food Administration to bridge the gap between centralized planning and decentralized execution of those plans, so would they now serve as a means for resolving the tension between Hoover's elitism and his commitment to the democratic ethos.

One might note, in fact, that Hoover's high regard for publicity, his belief in the efficacy of mobilizing public opinion to effect large public policies, and his view of the journalist, editor, magazine, and newspaper as "partners" in the work of the policy-maker,[61] all attitudes that he had held as early as his work for the Panama-Pacific Exposition, were also typical progressive attitudes. As several historians have noted, the progressive period placed a high value on popular education and social reform through journalism. Both Theodore Roosevelt and Woodrow Wilson appreciated the uses to which publicity might be put in carrying out social reforms, and both conceived of its deployment via the press as part of a process of "educational leadership."[62] Reform journalism, in the words of Rush Welter, was an important "informal device" in the progressive movement's attempt "to find ways of educating the self-governing public to a better understanding of contemporary problems."[63] Or, as Richard Hofstadter has put it:

To an extraordinary degree the work of the Progressive movement rested upon its journalism. The fundamental critical achievement of American Progressivism was the business of exposure, and journalism was the chief occupational source of its creative writers. It is hardly an exaggeration to say that the Progressive mind was characteristically a journalistic mind, and that its characteristic contribution was that of the socially responsible reporter-reformer. The muckraker was a central figure. Before there could be action, there must be information and exhortation. Grievances had to be given specific objects, and these the muckraker supplied. It was muckraking that brought the diffuse malaise of the public into focus.[64]

Thus, running through much of progressivism was the conviction that educating "the people" through the mass media would enable them to handle social problems without sacrificing democratic ideals. And it was this conviction that Hoover carried into the 1920s and acted upon to a greater extent than any other public official. Through the deployment of his public relations machinery and the utilization of his many press contacts, he became America's foremost public "instructor" in the "new era."

Indeed, as one reflects upon Hoover's activities, rhetoric, and style, he is impressed by the extent to which the man regarded himself as a public "educator," a view that may have been shaped by his academic connections as well as his progressivism. Prior to entering public service, he had been an influential Stanford trustee, a lecturer in mining engineering at Columbia and Stanford, and an active member of several learned scientific societies, all positions in which he had formed close ties with institutions of higher education; and once in public life, he was careful to maintain and expand these ties.[65] In any event, his pose, rhetoric, and approach were often those of deeply concerned pedagogue. In 1914, it will be recalled, he had hoped that his work on behalf of the Panama-Pacific Exposition would "advance the education of [the American] people" in international affairs. In 1917, as food administrator, he had referred to his work as a process of "constant hammering and teaching," and had seen the propaganda of his "Education Division" as important in instructing the citizenry in proper nutrition as well as food conservation.[66] And in 1920, he commented that "only by propaganda" was "there any promise of educating the American public . . . in the ideals of democracy."[67] One must note, too, that many of his statements of the 1919-20 period resemble commencement addresses, particularly in their sweeping world-encompassing analyses of the role of the United States in the "new era" of rapid economic change and conflicting ideologies. In them, he explained to his audience the causes of such social phenomena as world conflict, rapid urbanization, and the Communist revolution, interpreted for them the meaning of such phenomena and their relation to developments in the United States, and drew "lessons" with which to guide future policy. Always, as he discussed such matters, Hoover's stance was that of the public lecturer and "educator," never that of the political campaigner.[68] Consequently when he became secretary of commerce, he continued to view his function as that of "an economic interpreter to the American people,"[69] as head of "a clearing house [for the] helpful dissemination of ideas,"[70] or of "a domestic intelligence department to inform the public as well as the men in trade and commerce."[71] And to aid in this task of "ceaseless public education on the elemental facts,"[72] to "insure that the community [acted out of] knowledge rather than in ignorance,"[73] he mobilized publicity and gladly accepted the assistance of his many friends in the press.

In view of the stock image of Hoover as a conservative business figure, it is also interesting to observe how many of the former muckrake journalists of the progressive period were either Hoover's fervent admirers or very close friends and supporters. In Hoover, these people evidently saw the ideal progressive leader—an intelligent, knowledgeable man selflessly committed to administering to the needs of society through public education. As Ray Stannard Baker, a close friend of Theodore Roosevelt and exponent of a number of reform causes, put it when Hoover returned from Europe in 1919, the former food administrator was

> just the kind of man we need in politics now in America, perhaps even in the very highest place. There are very few men who possess in such high degree the passion of disinterested service, combined with really great gifts of leadership. He is an able and skilled administrator, with years of training in large affairs. He has a thorough-going liberal spirit and would approach the new

economic and industrial problems confronting us, not only with practical knowledge, but with breadth of sympathy and truly progressive views. . . . There is no public man in America who knows every phase of the foreign situation as comprehensively as Herbert Hoover, and none who has been able to deal more skillfully with complicated international problems. No one who saw him in action at Paris can doubt either his knowledge of these conditions or his genius for dealing with them. . . . While he has a firm and practical grasp upon realities and knows well how to deal with them, he has not lost the intense spirit of American idealism. Finally, and perhaps best of all, he has unlimited courage.[74]

Baker's sentiments, moreover, were shared by a variety of other celebrated muckrakers. Ida Tarbell, well known for her muckraking exposure of the Standard Oil Company, had worked with Hoover as a publicist for the Food Administration and member of the President's Unemployment Conference of 1921, which Hoover had convened and chaired. She fully appreciated his "enormous skills" and viewed him in 1922 as "the only person . . . in Washington [with] the will and openminded[ness] to understand the problems of the suffering and the uneducated."[75] Will Irwin, Hoover's fast friend and sometime publicist (both officially and unofficially), had been a managing editor for the muckraking *McClure's* magazine[76] and had contributed muckraking articles to *Collier's*,[77] then edited by Norman Hapgood. Hapgood himself, as his correspondence with Hoover reveals, was yet another great admirer of Hoover;[78] and Mark Sullivan, also associated with *Collier's*, became Hoover's friend and next door neighbor in Washington, an editor for his *American Individualism* and adviser on his speeches, and a privileged member of the "medicine ball cabinet" during the presidential years.[79] In addition, William Hard, a lesser-known muckraker before the war, became a close friend of Hoover in the 1920s (he too would become a member of the "medicine ball cabinet"), performed a great many publicity services for him,[80] and wrote a laudatory biography in 1928, celebrating his prodigious knowledge and his "educative and persuasive"[81] approach to government. And finally, there was William Allen White, still another Hoover companion and champion with a background in reform journalism and politics.[82]

In his rhetoric and social attitudes, his educational approach to the public, and his assumption that the scholar and the journalist were partners of the governmental executive in the making and promulgation of public policy, Hoover ought to be seen by historians today (as he was by many of his reformer friends and contemporaries) as a post-war survival of progressivism in the executive branch of government. It is true that as the 1920s passed by Hoover's fear of the federal government's actively intervening in the economy deepened. So great was this fear that he came to view federal legislation itself—even simply regulatory legislation—as, at best, inefficient and, at worst, tending to bureaucratic domination by the national state. But his grave concern here was not the product of a probusiness orientation as some have assumed; it was rather a concern that he shared with many progressives, and one that stemmed from his wartime apprehension of what bureaucracy could do to democratic institutions and values.[83] While acclaiming the journalistic exposures and the legislative reforms of the progressive era, he was convinced that the federal government had been sufficiently strengthened to prevent domination by big business.[84] What was needed now was not further legislative solutions but solutions reached through demobilization of the wartime state—solutions dependent upon the "education and voluntary action of our people."[85] The role of government in the "new era" was not to "cure foolishness by legislation" or to "catch an economic force with a policeman" or a "bureau."[86] Rather, it should function to educate, disseminate information, and create cooperation between groups in order to promote the welfare and growth of the whole social and economic order.[87] Nor were such doctrines an excuse for inaction, as they were with some conservatives. Hoover was indefatigable in trying to organize cooperation and make his approach work.

To govern without resorting to legislation, to utilize the expertise of the scientist, economist, and businessman in tandem with the resources of local communities and private institutions, to achieve social and economic stability while preserving democratic institutions and values—these, as Hoover saw it, were the central problems. And one way to solve them was through the mobilization and proper use of publicity. As he had once campaigned in the press for the Panama-Pacific Exposition, for Belgium, and for wartime food conservation, so would he campaign via the mass media of the 1920s for a multitude of domestic social and economic causes designed to advance social progress while forestalling the growth of big government. Thus, his social outlook and political philosophy led to an approach quite similar to the one demanded by the ambivalent, aggressive, yet introverted, nature of his personality. The two, in effect, reinforced and combined with each other. His behind the scenes apolitical administrative posture fused with his negative attitudes toward the role of the state. His personal desire for influence merged with his great concern for social control and guidance. And together, they produced an extraordinary reliance upon publicity as an administrative tool, one that stemmed both from psychological needs and intellectual commitments. It is an index to the depth of bitterness and frustration engendered by the depression that so many independent journalists should fail to recognize this fact and instead ascribe Hoover's use of publicity to an overweening ambition for the presidency.

1.   As recently as 1969, a student of the 1930s has written: "Herbert Clark Hoover . . . was as deeply imbued with Quaker morality as with faith in the economic philosophy of laissez-faire" (Cabell Phillips, *From the Crash to the Blitz, 1929-1939* [New York, 1969], p. 41).

2.   John D. Hicks, *Republican Ascendancy, 1920-1933*, p. 202. Even relatively sympathetic interpreters of Hoover's career have viewed him as a Social Darwinist. See, for example, Harris G. Warren, *Herbert Hoover and the Great Depression*, p. 33, and Richard Hofstadter, *The American Political Tradition*, pp. 294-98. Although Hofstadter recognizes Hoover's "allegiance to progressivism," he feels Hoover's commitment "to the abstract principle of laissez-faire" was the more important ingredient in his social thought.

3.   Herbert Hoover, "Food Administration," Address Before the National Chamber of Commerce Convention, September 19, 1917, 4-A, Public Statements, HHP, HHPL.

4.   During his years of travel and residence abroad, Hoover had become, through reading and direct observation, a perceptive student of the many countries he visited—especially China and Russia. At a time when China was appealing

to many Americans as a great potential market and as a land moving heroically toward democracy, he realized that both these views were false. His personal experiencing of the "hideous social and governmental" situation in Russia in 1910 led him to believe that the "country could blow up some day" (Herbert Hoover, *The Memoirs of Herbert Hoover, 1874-1920: The Years of Adventure*, 1:67, 71-72, 105). When the war broke out, Hoover was aware of what it meant for the "modern, intricate, economic world." He experienced it as an "earthquake. . . . The substance and bottom seemed to go out of everything" (ibid., p. 140). Yet for all his analytical acumen in comprehending the Chinese and Russian societies and the consequences of the war upon the west, he had not forseen the coming of the war itself—even within days of the German attack through Belgium. Like many others, he had misunderstood—and at the time he composed his *Memoirs*, still misunderstood—Norman Angell's argument in his widely read *The Great Illusion* (1909). In his misreading, he was persuaded by the book that the financial interdependence of Europe would make war impossible (ibid., p. 138). The thrust of Angell's argument, however, was not that financial interdependence meant the end of war; he was contending rather that the state of financial interdependence simply meant that there could be no longer any winners in war (Norman Angell, *After All: The Autobiography of Norman Angell*, pp. 150-54).

5. Hoover, *Memoirs*, 1:135.

6. Ibid., pp. 135-36.

7. Hoover to Frederick R. Coudert, November 2, 1918, 11, Public Statements (the letter in which these phrases occur was printed in the New York *Times*), HHP, HHPL.

8. Hoover to All Representatives of the Food Administration, November 12, 1918, 11-A, Public Statements, HHP, HHPL.

9. Herbert Hoover, "The European Food Situation," U.S. Food Administration Official Statement No. 8, November 6, 1918, 11-C, Public Statements, HHP, HHPL.

10. Herbert Hoover, "The Food Situation in Liberated Territories," 13 Public Statements, HHP, HHPL.

11. Herbert Hoover, "The Food Future: What Every American Mouthful Means to Europe," 14, Public Statements, HHP, HHPL.

12. Herbert Hoover, "Why We Are Feeding Germany," Press Statement, March 21, 1919, 16, Public Statements, HHP, HHPL; "Starvation in Europe," Press Statement, December 17, 1919, 38-A, Public Statements, HHP, HHPL.

13. Hoover, "Without a League of Nations to Guide New Republics Europe Will Go Back to Chaos," N.Y. *Times*, July 28, 1919, 21-C, Public Statements, HHP, HHPL; "Economic, Social, and Industrial Problems Confronting the Nation: The Maintenance of Our National Ideals," 55-A, Public Statements, HHP, HHPL.

14. Hoover, Address at the Chevy Chase Club, July 10, 1917, 3-B, Public Statements, HHP, HHPL.

15. Hoover, "Conserving the Food Supply," 3-F, Public Statements, HHP, HHPL.

16. Hoover, "Food Administration," Address Delivered at National Chamber of Commerce, September 19, 1917, 4-A, Public Statements, HHP, HHPL.

17. Hoover, *Memoirs*, 1:245; Hoover, Address at the Chevy Chase Club, July 10, 1917, 3-B, Public Statements, HHP, HHPL.

18. Herbert Hoover, *The Memoirs of Herbert Hoover: The Cabinet and the Presidency, 1920-1933*, 2:28.

19. Ibid., p. 2; Press Statement on Future Plans upon Return to California, September 27, 1919, 26, Public Statements, HHP, HHPL; Hoover, *Memoirs*, 2:4.

20. Ray Lyman Wilbur to Edgar Rickard, September 29, 1919, Ray Lyman Wilbur Papers, "Political—1920"; George Barr Baker to Hoover, December 2 and 3, 1919, George Barr Baker Papers, Box 3, Hoover Institution on War, Revolution, and Peace.

21. Hoover, *Memoirs*, 2:4.

22. Herbert Hoover, "Self-Expression Is the Need of Today," *Business Methods*, November, 1920, 100-A, Public Statements, HHP, HHPL.

23. Hoover, Address Delivered before American Institute of Mining Engineers, August 26, 1920, 84, Public Statements, HHP, HHPL.

24. Hoover, Foreword to *America and the New Era*, by M. Friedman, February 4, 1920, 42-A, Public Statements, HHP, HHPL.

25. When he began his work as secretary of commerce, Hoover secured the services of academic economists Edwin F. Gay and Wesley Mitchell. Gay became an "expert consultant" to the department and as a member of the National Bureau of Economic Research was involved in the preparation of the report on business cycles and unemployment undertaken by the bureau in 1921-22 at Hoover's request (Herbert Heaton, *A Scholar in Action: Edwin F. Gay*, pp. 188-91). Hoover had wanted Mitchell to serve as an "economic adviser to the entire Department." Mitchell, though gratified at the secretary's "effort to make use of whatever economics can render to government," turned him down. However, as director of the National Bureau of Economic Research, he cooperated fully with Hoover on the business cycle and unemployment study (Hoover to Wesley C. Mitchell, July 29, 1921; Mitchell to Hoover, August 3, 1921, Secretary of Commerce Official File, "Mitchell, Wesley," HHP, HHPL). Hoover's elitist views—which necessitated the recruitment of experts such as Gay and Mitchell—emerge strongly in the following passage of his book *American Individualism* (1922): "Our social, economic and intellectual progress is almost solely dependent upon the creative minds of those individuals with imaginative and administrative intelligence who create or who carry discoveries to widespread application. No race possesses more than a small percentage of these minds in a single generation. . . . Acts and ideas that lead to progress are born out of the womb of the individual mind, not out of the mind of the crowd. The crowd only feels; it has no mind of its own which can plan. The crowd is credulous, it destroys, it consumes, it hates, and it dreams—but it never builds. . . . The demagogue feeds on mob emotions and his leadership is the leadership of emotion, not the leadership of intellect and progress. Popular desires are no criteria to the real need; they [*sic*] can be determined only by deliberate consideration, by education, by constructive leadership" (pp. 22-25).

26. P. 3.

27. Hoover, Address at Dinner Given in His Honor by the American Institute of Mining and Metallurgical Engineers, September 16, 1919, 25, Public Statements, HHP, HHPL.

28. Hoover, *Memoirs*, 2:v.

29. Herbert Hoover, "Economic, Social, and Industrial Problems Confronting the Nation: The Maintenance of Our National Ideals," 55-A, Public Statements, HHP, HHPL.

30. Ibid.; "Some Phases of American Idealism," Address at Methodist Conference, April 9, 1920, 57, Public Statements, HHP, HHPL; "Some Notes on Industrial Readjustment," 39, Public Statements, HHP, HHPL; Foreword to *America*

and the New Era by M. Friedman, February 4, 1920, 42-A, Public Statements, HHP, HHPL.

31. Hoover, Address at Dinner Given in His Honor by American Institute of Mining and Metallurgical Engineers, September 16, 1919, 25, Public Statements, HHP, HHPL; Address before the San Francisco Commercial Club, October 9, 1919, 28, Public Statements, HHP, HHPL; "The Paramount Business of Every American Today," 76, Public Statements, HHP, HHPL.

32. Herbert Hoover, "Neighborhood (Settlement) Houses Help Solve Social Problems," 74, Public Statements, HHP, HHPL.

33. Hoover, Penn College Commencement Address, June 12, 1925, 496, Public Statements, HHP, HHPL.

34. Hoover, "Views on Bolshevism," Press Statement, April 25, 1919, 19, Public Statements, HHP, HHPL; Address Given in His Honor by American Institute of Mining and Metallurgical Engineers, September 16, 1919, 25, Public Statements, HHP, HHPL; "Some Notes on Industrial Readjustment," 39, Public Statements, HHP, HHPL.

35. Hoover, Address at Dinner in His Honor by American Institute of Mining and Metallurgy, September 16, 1919, 25, Public Statements, HHP, HHPL.

36. Hoover, Address before Methodist Conference, April 9, 1920, 57, Public Statements, HHP, HHPL.

37. Hoover, "Economic, Social, and Industrial Problems Confronting the Nation: The Maintenance of Our National Ideals," 55-A, Public Statements, HHP, HHPL.

38. Hoover, "Food Administration in Relation to the Farmer," Address before the Conference of Editors and Publishers of Farm Papers, August 25, 1917, 3-J, Public Statements, HHP, HHPL; "Food Administration," Address before the National Chamber of Commerce Convention, September 19, 1917, 4-A, Public Statements, HHP, HHPL.

39. Hoover, *Memoirs*, 1:244, 252.

40. John D. Hicks's interpretation of Hoover as representing "the industrialists' point of view" and embodying "the single-interest [business] domination under which the Republican party had fallen" by 1928 may be taken as a fairly typical "liberal" historical appraisal of Hoover (John D. Hicks, *Republican Ascendancy, 1921-1933*, pp. 202, 208). So-called new left historians William Appleman Williams and Barton J. Bernstein have challenged this conventional and still largely accepted view by asserting Hoover's progressivism: William A. Williams, *The Contours of American History* (Chicago, 1961), pp. 426-27; Barton J. Bernstein, "The New Deal: The Conservative Achievements of Liberal Reform," in Bernstein, ed., *Towards a New Past: Dissenting Essays in American History*, p. 266. Looking at Hoover from the opposite political pole, Murray N. Rothbard has arrived at the same point of view (Murray N. Rothbard, *America's Great Depression* [Princeton, N.J., 1963], pp. 167-85. Recognition of the inadequacy of the standard view point may also be found in Carl Degler "The Ordeal of Herbert Hoover," pp. 563-83, and George Edwin Mowry, *The Urban Nation*, pp. 56-63.

41. In a 1922 assessment of the role of the engineer in public life, Hoover wrote: "This great body of men in administrative and technical service penetrates every industrial avenue and thus possesses a unique understanding of many of our intricate economic problems and an influence in their solution not equalled by any other part of the community. Wanting nothing from the public either individually

or collectively they are in a position of disinterested service" (SCOF, "Feiker, 1921-1922," HHP, HHPL).

42.   William Allen White, *The Autobiography of William Allen White*, p. 486; Hoover, *Memoirs*, 1:120.

43.   George E. Mowry, *The California Progressives*, pp. 13, 19, 29, 23-24, 130; Ann Lane and Louise H. Wall, eds., *The Letters of Franklin K. Lane* (New York, 1922), p. 163.

44.   Ray Lyman Wilbur, *The Memoirs of Ray Lyman Wilbur, 1875-1949*, p. 256.

45.   C. C. Regier, *The Era of the Muckrakers*, pp. 150, 154, 161, 166-69.

46.   *Who's Who in America, 1930-1931*, 16 (Chicago, 1930): 225; Regier, *The Era of the Muckrakers*, pp. 142-43.

47.   "The Secretariat," *American Mercury*, 18 (December, 1929): 392-93; [Drew Pearson], *Washington Merry-Go-Round* (New York, 1931), pp. 308-9; John Chamberlain, *Farewell to Reform: The Rise, Life and Decay of the Progressive Mind in America* (New York, 1932), p. 129.

48.   Hoover to Ralph Arnold, March 8, 1920, 50, Public Statements (Letter Published in the Balitimore *Sun*, New York *Times*, and New York *Tribune*), HHP, HHPL.

49.   Hoover, "America's Obligations in Belgium Relief," Address before the Chamber of Commerce of New York State, February 1, 1917, 1, Public Statements, HHP, HHPL; "Bind the Wounds of France," 1-C, Public Statements, HHP, HHPL. Hoover's subscription to "reform Darwinism" is explicit in his view of the nature of the war: "We have entered upon a war entirely unique in its character in that it is a war against ideas. The German people have adopted the theory of the survival of the strongest, the right of might, a biological interpretation of the theory of evolution, without any of that fine tempering which the Anglo-Saxon race has included in its sociological application through the belief that civilization spells the protection of the helpless" ("Conserving the Food Supply," 3-F, Public Statements, HHP, HHPL).

50.   Richard Hofstadter, in characterizing the social outlook of the prewar progressives, has written: "Representing as they did the spirit and desires of the middle class, the Progressives stood for a dual program of economic remedies designed to minimize the dangers from the extreme left and right.   On one side they feared the power of the plutocracy, on the other the poverty and restlessness of the masses" (Richard Hofstadter, *The Age of Reform*, p. 238).

51.   Hoover, Milwaukee Speech on Behalf of Senator Lenroot, August 31, 1920, 84-A, Public Statements, HHP, HHPL.

52.   Hoover, Address before the Federated American Engineering Societies, November 18, 1920, 102, Public Statements, HHP, HHPL.

53.   Ibid.

54.   Ibid.

55.   Ibid.; Hoover's labor position was actually more advanced and enlightened than that of many prewar progressives who in Mowry's words had been "emotionally . . . more opposed to collectivism from below . . . than above" (George Edwin Mowry, *The Era of Theodore Roosevelt*, p. 100). His conviction that management and government had to recognize labor's bargaining rights if social stability was ever to be achieved is traceable as far back as his junior year in college. His reaction to the government's handling of the Pullman workers' and American Railway Union strike is given in a letter of July, 1894: "I suppose you have seen the

strike. I also have been doing some laboratory work in political economy. I was tied up between San Francisco, Oakland, and Sacramento for three weeks and so have seen much of it. I rather think it is a sort of boil on the "body politic" that has been driven back into the system by the U.S. and which will come out worse next time" (Hoover to an unknown correspondent, July 19, 1894, Pre-Commerce Correspondence, HHP, HHPL). In his lectures on mining engineering given in 1909, he had observed: "As corporations have grown, so likewise have the labor unions. In general, they are normal and proper antidotes for unlimited capitalistic organization. . . . The time when the employer could ride roughshod over his labor is disappearing with the doctrine of 'laissez faire' on which it was founded. The sooner the fact is recognized, the better for the employer" (Herbert Hoover, *Principles of Mining*, pp. 167-68).

56. Hoover, Address before the Federated American Engineering Societies, November 18, 1920, 102; Public Statements, HHP, HHPL.

57. Ibid.

58. Hoover, Address before the Associated Charities of San Francisco, December 29, 1919, 40, Public Statements, HHP, HHPL; Address before the Cleveland Community Chest Organization, November 15, 1920, 101, Public Statements, HHP, HHPL; Foreword to *America and the New Era* by M. Friedman, February 4, 1920, 42-A, Public Statements, HHP, HHPL; "A Program for American Children," Address before the American Child Hygiene Association, October 11, 1920, 93, Public Statements, HHP, HHPL; "Neighborhood (Settlement) Houses Help Solve Social Problem," HHP, HHPL; "Economic, Social, and Industrial Problems Confronting the Nation: The Maintenance of Our National Ideals," 55-A, Public Statements, HHP, HHPL; "The Purpose of '*Better Times*'," Advertisement for *Better Times* December, 1920, 108-A, Public Statements, HHP, HHPL.

59. Quoted in Alpheus Thomas Mason, *Brandeis: A Free Man's Life*, p. 530; Frank W. Taussig to Hoover, February 3, 1920, Pre-Commerce Correspondence, HHP, HHPL; Letter quoted in Edward A. Ross, *Seventy Years of It*, p. 236.

60. Frederick Jackson Turner, progressive historian, found the views expressed in his *The Frontier in American History* (1920) confirmed by Hoover's "meaty little book on American Individualism"—"a book written by a statesman and man of large affairs, approaching the subject in an independent way" (Frederick Jackson Turner to Richard S. Emmet, a Hoover secretary, January 18, 1923, SCPF, "Turner, Frederick Jackson," HHP, HHPL). Edwin R. Seligman, like Taussig a reform-minded economist, wrote Hoover that though he "knew well of [Hoover's] accomplishments as a statesman and a professional man," he had had "no idea that [he] was so erudite a scholar" until he had read Hoover's translation of Agricola's treatise on mining (Edwin R. Seligman to Hoover, December 24, 1924, SCPF, "Seligman, Edwin R.," HHP, HHPL). Walter Lippmann expressed his admiration for Hoover's work on several occasions. He may have seen in Hoover his "innovator in politics," for he once asked him for his cooperation in writing an article for the *Atlantic Monthly* on "the place of the scientifically trained man in our political system" (Walter Lippmann to Hoover, January 7, 1922; September 29, 1922; July 15, 1925, SCOF, "Lippmann, Walter," HHP, HHPL).

61. In his foreword to Friedman's *America and the New Era*, Hoover wrote: "The motivating influence to progress has been the American social conscience. The ethics of big business have risen since 1900 . . . as a result of the awakening of the conscience of America. In the matter of trusts, railways, tariff and rural credits, there has been increasing public condemnation of pillage in high places and a corresponding extra-juridical submission to public opinion. Our industrial development

has outrun legal procedure and the lag is made less hurtful to the community because of the power of public opinion, a force more potent and pervasive than the law itself" (42-A, Public Statements, HHP, HHPL). Hoover recognized the influence that publicists for reform such as Theodore Roosevelt and novelist Frank Norris had had in "awakening the national conscience" and correcting social abuses (Address at Conference of Representatives of Grain Trade of the United States with the Food Administration Grain Corporation, April 30, 1918, 7, Public Statements, HHP, HHPL; "Tribute to Theodore Roosevelt," Address at Rocky Mountain Club Dinner, October 27, 1919, 30, Public Statements, HHP, HHPL). Hoover regarded his journalist friends as "public servants" joined in the "effort to promote public good" (Statement on Death of Melville E. Stone, February 16, 1929, 975, Public Statements, HHP, HHPL; Hoover to Frederick Wile, June 5, 1922, SCPF, "Wile, Frederick," HHP, HHPL).

62. Rush Welter, *Popular Education and Democratic Thought in America*, pp. 250-57; Eric F. Goldman, *Two-Way Street: The Emergence of the Public Relations Counsel*, p. 5.

63. *Popular Education and Democratic Thought in America*, p. 250.

64. *The Age of Reform*, pp. 186-87.

65. Will Irwin has noted that Hoover's love for his *alma mater*, Stanford University, was so strong that it "became a kind of complex" with him (Will Irwin, *Herbert Hoover: A Reminiscent Biography*, p. 44). In the years after his graduation, he contributed books and money to the university and became a distingushed member of the Stanford chapter of Sigma Xi, a national scientific society that undertook original investigations in pure and applied science (David Starr Jordan, *The Days of a Man*, 2:206; Wilbur, *The Memoirs of Ray Lyman Wilbur*, pp. 132, 210). In 1912, he became a trustee of the university and was instrumental in bringing about the ascension of his old mentor and friend Dr. John Branner to the presidency of the institution in 1913 (Jordan, *The Days of a Man*, pp. 455-58). In 1915, Hoover helped his friend and former classmate Ray Lyman Wilbur succeed to the presidency. He later tapped Wilbur to head the Food Administration's Food Conservation Division and, when president, the Department of the Interior. When he returned from Europe in 1919, he built what would become his permanent residence on the Stanford campus. Throughout the 1920s, he remained close to Stanford affairs through Wilbur, and in 1924 and 1925, he was the prime mover in the creation of Stanford's Graduate School of Business Administration. Long concerned with the professionalization of the engineer and the businessman, in 1925, Hoover was also associated with Harvard's pioneering Graduate School of Business in an advisory capacity (Hoover to Wallace B. Donham, dean of Harvard Graduate School of Business Administration, December 8, 1925, SCPF, "Donham, Wallace B.," HHP, HHPL). Many of Hoover's friends and associates in his Commerce Department work, e.g., Arch Shaw, Frederick Feiker, Wesley Mitchell, and Edwin F. Gay, had been involved in the organization of the Harvard Graduate School of Business and had offered courses within it (Melvin T. Copeland, *And Mark an Era: The Story of the Harvard Business School*, pp. 343-64; "Feiker, Frederick," *Who's Who in America, 1932-33* 17 [Chicago, 1932]: p. 818). Given these close associations to the academic community and his distaste for politics, Hoover may not have been entirely in jest when he confided to Gay in 1922 that he "wished he were a professor" (Heaton, *Edwin F. Gay: A Scholar in Action*, p. 191).

66. Shortly after he became food administrator, Hoover wrote President Wilson: "We are engaged in organizing a definite course of instruction in all of the schools, primary as well as secondary, on nutrition and food economics generally.

We are having the fine cooperation of the Bureau of Education in the preparation and distribution of a series of textbooks on this subject. . . ."

"We feel that, by taking advantage of the war emotion, we here have an opportunity of introducing intelligibly into the minds of the children, not only fundamental data on nutrition, but also of being able to secure its permanent inclusion in school curricula, and, therefore, feel that it is a matter of more than ordinary propaganda importance" (Hoover to Woodrow Wilson, August 21, 1917, Pre-Commerce Correspondence, HHP, HHPL).

67. Hoover, Address before the Food Conference of Pennsylvania Public Safety Committee, September 29, 1917, 4-B, Public Statements, HHP, HHPL; Address at the Northwestern Miller Dinner, August 21, 1920, 82, Public Statements, HHP, HHPL.

68. On this point see especially, Hoover, "Views on Bolshevism," Press Statement, April 25, 1919, 19, Public Statements, HHP, HHPL; Address at Dinner Given in His Honor by the A.I.M.M.E., September 16, 1919, 25, Public Statements, HHP, HHPL; Address before the San Francisco Commercial Club, October 9, 1919, 28, Public Statements, HHP, HHPL; "Some Notes on Industrial Readjustment," 39, Public Statements, HHP, HHPL; Penn College Commencement Address, June 12, 1925, 496, Public Statements, HHP, HHPL; "Problems of Our Economic Development," Address to Stanford University Seniors, June 22, 1925, 499, Public Statements, HHP, HHPL.

69. Hoover to Wesley C. Mitchell, July 29, 1921, "Mitchell, Wesley C.," HHP, HHPL; *Ninth Annual Report of the Secretary of Commerce* (Washington, 1921), p. 6.

70. Hoover, "Cooperation between Shippers and Railways," Letter to National and State Trade Associations (Published in New York *Times* and *Commercial and Financial Chronicle*), April 1, 1923, 303-A, Public Statements, HHP, HHPL.

71. Hoover, "Facing Our Economic Facts," 166, Public Statements, HHP, HHPL. Hoover evidently saw himself not only as teacher to the nation but also, in a very concrete sense, as an instructor to his Department of Commerce subordinates. Throughout his tenure as commerce secretary, he held weekly Saturday morning conferences with his bureau chiefs and their subordinates. These conferences were called for no other reason than to keep his staff abreast of current events at home and abroad and to point out the relevance of the department's varied tasks to those events. The "method of instruction" was one of questioning an appropriate staff member about an issue and then opening the subject up for general discussion (SCOF, "Secretary's Conferences, 1922-1927," HHP, HHPL). Reflecting upon the large number of his staff who had departed for work in business and industry, Hoover once observed proudly that the department was "a post graduate school of American life" and that it was "attaining a fair sized alumni association" (Speech at Dinner Given in Honor of Secretary and Mrs. Hoover by Employees of the Department of Commerce, March 9, 1925, 452, Public Statements, HHP, HHPL).

72. Hoover, "Relation of the Electric Railway Industry in Industrial Efficiency," Speech Before the American Electric Railway Association, October 6, 1921, 176, Public Statements, HHP, HHPL.

73. Hoover, Address before the Trade Association Conference, April 12, 1922, 220, Public Statements, HHP, HHPL.

74. From a clipping in the Springfield *Republican*, September 17, 1919, which Baker sent to Hoover. Ray Stannard Baker to Hoover, September, 1919, Pre-Commerce Correspondence, HHP, HHPL.

75. Ida Tarbell, *All in the Day's Work: An Autobiography*, pp. 321, 375; Ida Tarbell to Hoover, October 12, 1922, SCPF, "Tarbell, Ida," HHP, HHPL.

76. Will Irwin, *The Making of a Reporter*, pp. 129-30.

77. Ibid., pp. 137-38; see for example, Irwin's "The First Ward Ball," anthologized in Arthur and Lila Weinberg, eds., *The Muckrakers*, pp. 139-45.

78. Hapgood to Hoover, n.d. 19, 1920, and July 28, 1920, Pre-Commerce Correspondence, HHP, HHPL; Hapgood to Hoover, October 2, 1923, and February 13, 1924, SCPF, "Hapgood, Norman," HHP, HHPL.

79. Mark Sullivan, *The Education of an American*, pp. 316-17; Regier, *The Era of the Muckrakers*, pp. 103, 119, 138, 181; Hoover to Sullivan, September 27, 1921, Mark Sullivan Collection, Box 14, Hoover Institution on War, Revolution, and Peace. Sullivan to Hoover, October 13, 1921, SCOF; Sullivan to Hoover, April 26, 1926; Sullivan to George Akerson, April 12, 1927, SCPF, HHP, HHPL. Late in his presidency, Hoover noted in answer to a letter from a member of the League for Political Education that in his opinion Sullivan was the American writer "best qualified to mould the thinking of the American people" (French Strother to President of the League for Political Education, February 6, 1933, Presidential Papers, White House Secretaries File—French Strother Files, HHP, HHPL).

80. Hard, a correspondent for the *Nation* and contributor to many other magazines and newspapers, publicized Hoover's views on subjects ranging from the Colorado River project and the conservation of American fishing resources to American education and the development of federal controls for the radio industry. He once represented Hoover's position on the radio controls question against that of his own employer, Oswald Garrison Villard, editor of the *Nation*. Through the medium of radio, he further communicated Hoover's points of view to the public. Information for his speeches and articles derived from interviews with Hoover and materials supplied from Hoover's office. Hoover had a high regard for Hard's "delicacy of touch, appreciation of serious and difficult questions, . . . and illuminative lucidity" (Hoover to Hard, March 4, 1924, SCOF and SCPF, "William Hard," HHP, HHPL).

81. William Hard, *Who's Hoover?*, p. 191; Regier, *The Era of the Muckrakers*, pp. 191, 131, 154, 212. Two of Hard's muckraking pieces in *Collier's* and *Everybody's* are anthologized in the Weinbergs' *The Muckrakers, 1902-1912*, pp. 87-98, 342-58.

82. White was in frequent communication with Hoover throughout the 1920s. In 1923, he elicited from Hoover a lengthy statement deploring the threat of "bloc government" to the two-party American system of government. He published this statement in his Emporia *Daily Gazette* and the New York *Times* (Hoover to William Allen White, December 28, 1923, SCPF, "White, William Allen," HHP, HHPL; 343, Public Statements, HHP, HHPL). In the spring of 1927, he arranged an informal dinner for Hoover and some fifty to seventy-five Kansas newspaper editors (White to Hoover, May 12, 1927, SCPF, "White, William Allen," HHP, HHPL). Arthur Capper, progressive senator from Kansas, editor of the *Topeka Daily Capital*, and also a personal friend of Hoover, editorialized in his paper: "This meeting of Kansas editors was an ovation to Mr. Hoover, the handy-man of America. He was the target for many questions on flood control, waterway development, superpower, installment buying, aviation, [and other] economic problems. . . . Hearing Herbert Hoover in a familiar and intimate talk on economic problems leaves the feeling that this country is making some progress towards government by engineers and science, instead of by lawyers and vested interests" (July 19, 1927, SCPF, "White, William Allen," HHP, HHPL). White was one of the first editors George

Akerson called upon to help "mould public sentiment" behind Hoover's candidacy for the presidency in 1928 (George Akerson to White, October 10, 1927, George E. Akerson Papers, HHPL). White did write propaganda for Hoover during the campaign.

83. In a comprehensive study of the reactions of the older progressives to the New Deal (a well-defined group of 168 former reformers), Otis Graham has found that approximately 60 percent opposed the New Deal for the following reasons: a war-wrought fear of the state, a distaste for the New Deal's "class" and "materialistic" orientation, its lack of traditional philosophical underpinnings, a personal dislike for Franklin D. Roosevelt's political style, and a nostalgia for a decentralized, agrarian past. Though these were Hoover's reasons and though Graham recognizes that opposition to the New Deal was strongest among "the journalist-editor group" of the old progressives (many of whom were Hoover's friends), Graham, in an oversight common among liberal historians, persists in seeing Hoover, not as an old progressive, but as a "dedicated proponent of things as they are," "an outraged constitutionalist," and a member of the "reactionary wing" of the Republican party (Otis Graham, *An Encore for Reform: The Old Progressives and the New Deal*, pp. 24-100, 37, 66, 93).

84. Hoover, *American Individualism*, pp. 52-54.

85. "America and You," 60-A, Public Statements, HHP, HHPL.

86. "Important Issues before the Republican Convention," New York *Tribune* and Washington *Herald*, April 27, 1920, 60, Public Statements, HHP, HHPL; "Problems of Our Economic Evolution," Address to the Stanford University Seniors, June 22, 1925, 499, Public Statements, HHP, HHPL.

87. "What America Faces," 141, Public Statements, HHP, HHPL; Address before the Eleventh Annual Meeting of the Chamber of Commerce of the United States, 306, Public Statements, HHP, HHPL.

6 The Administrator as Publicist

WITH HIS CURIOUSLY CONFLICTING personality traits of assertiveness and passivity, Herbert Hoover, though anxious to exert public influence, had never rushed toward opportunities for "public service." As we have seen, he had been uncertain about accepting the CRB and Food Administration positions and had resisted the efforts of those who wanted to make him an authentic presidential candidate in 1920. When approached by President-elect Harding about a place in his cabinet late in 1920, he again hesitated.[1] But, as in the past, once he had overcome his doubts, he knew exactly what he wanted and moved boldly to achieve it.

Along with the Department of Commerce, Harding held out to him the historically more prestigious and powerful Department of the Interior. Hoover chose the former. Its enabling act, he found, constituted a "wide-open charter" for his principal concern, "the development and reconstruction" of the national economy;[2] and to guarantee that he would be able to exercise influence in all the areas specified—something, he felt, his predecessors had not done —he insisted, as a condition of acceptance, that he be given "a voice in all important economic policies of the administration." Harding and the other cabinet members agreed,[3] which meant that even before assuming office, Hoover had won for himself a large measure of power. With it, he hoped to meet the many challenges to American social and economic stability that he had identified in his speeches and articles of the immediate postwar period.

Hoover's initial press release as secretary of commerce, the first of hundreds issued by his Press Bureau to inform the public of his department's affairs,[4] constituted both a summation of his many messages of the two preceding years and a prologue to the public relations–oriented policies he was about to pursue. In it, he reiterated the major economic problems confronting the country, those of industrial inefficiency and waste, stagnating domestic and foreign trade, inadequate housing, widespread unemployment, and labor-management conflict. These, he continued, were the problems upon which his department would focus; and in seeking solutions it would emphasize "cooperation" with "industry," "trade," and the "community," not regulation of them. Its "expansion of governmental activity . . . would be in the constructive study and ventilation of the whole gamut" of America's economic ills.[5] And having investigated "economic questions," as he put it in a later report, it would secure action by pointing out "the remedy for economic failure or the road to progress," and by inspiring and assisting in "cooperative action" among all groups in the economy.[6] As in his previous administrative undertakings, Hoover would labor behind the scenes, relying heavily on publicity and public relations to "stimulate action among industries, trades, and consumers themselves."[7]

At the tactical level, this program for "national reconstruction and development" embraced a number of "campaigns" waged against particular problem areas in the economy. One of the most important of these, one that, in effect, constituted the leitmotif of Hoover's whole program, was the campaign to eliminate "national industrial waste," which, as conceived by Hoover, would "raise American standards of living" while avoiding "regulation and laws."[8] The seeds for this lay in the simplification and standardization work done by the Conservation Division of the War Industries Board during World War I.[9] At war's end, the division's functions, minus its coercive powers, had been transferred to the Department of Commerce, and since Arch Shaw, the man who had administered the work, was a close friend of Hoover, the latter early became intrigued with what a similar approach could accomplish in peacetime.[10] The war, he felt, with its need for "maximum production" had opened "a great vista of possibilities" in the direction of industrial standardization.[11] Accordingly, as president of the Federated American Engineering Societies in 1920 and 1921, he had instigated the preparation of a report, *Waste in Industry*, which was subsequently edited and publicized by Edward Hunt, and which found in simplification the best means to lower production costs and thus broaden domestic markets.[12] It was this report that underlay his campaign against waste, and shortly after his inauguration as secretary of commerce, he set out to implement its ideas by creating a Division of Simplified Practice in the Bureau of Standards.[13]

Under the direction of William A. Durgin, and after July, 1924, R. M. Hudson, the new division served as both an agency for "selling" the idea of simplification to American industry and one that would bring "producers and consumers together" for purposes of waste elimination.[14] Its activities were publicized, in part, through Donald Wilhelm's magazine articles, through such influential trade editors and "standardization experts" as Frederick Feiker and Arch Shaw,[15] and through the efforts of Ernest L. Priest of Lupton Wilkinson, Inc., who was hired in 1924 to write newspaper publicity, and who did succeed in placing material in hundreds of newspapers and trade journals in some 44 states and 205 cities.[16] Generally speaking, however, it was Durgin and Hudson, with their admirable "conceptions of public relations" and their ability to combine the qualities of "evangelist, educator, and salesman,"[17] who were most useful to Hoover. It was they who were responsible for the division's propagandistic *Monthly News Bulletin*, for hundreds of simplification speeches, and for scores of magazine articles, many of which were published in the trade journals presided over by Shaw and Feiker.[18]

Responding to this high-powered campaign, scores of industries, from paving brick manufacturers to milk bottle makers, sent representatives to the Commerce Department, where, in conference with their major consumers and with Hoover and his staff, they agreed to reduce drastically the styles and sizes of their products. Paving bricks, for instance, were reduced from 66 to 5 varieties, milk bottles from 49 to 9.[19] Then, as a follow-up to the conferences, Hoover made their recommendations and accomplishments the basis for additional publications and new press releases[20] and, in both 1925 and 1926, featured the simplification campaign in his *Annual Report* to the president.[21] This new publicity, in turn, brought more conferences, which generated more publicity and thus led to a steadily expanding movement. By mid-1927, it had produced 75 major simplifications, with 12 more in the planning stage, and had involved the cooperation of 898 trade associations and 6,676 individual firms.[22] Hoover claimed, moreover, that in reducing inventory and production costs and thus permitting lower prices, the crusade had saved "millions of dollars" for industry and the nation as a whole;[23] and, of major significance, it had required nothing beyond the use of publicity and conferences, demonstrating what government could do as a "friendly helper" rather than a "legislator" and "regulator."[24]

Hoover also made publicity an important administrative tool in "the fostering, promotion, and development of the foreign and domestic commerce of the United States." Sympathetic to the growing desire of businessmen for the sharing of statistical information among individual firms, a sharing that would inspire a "new competition" while providing stability,[25] he recommended to Congress that the government's statistical services "be vigorously expanded" to enable "the commercial public to judge the ebb and flow of economic currents."[26] Specifically, the Department of Commerce, as he envisioned it, should become "a real business information service to the country" and "an economic interpreter to the American public generally."[27] It should provide business executives with information pertaining to "the character and location of demand for their products," the "sources for labor and raw materials," the "credit and financial conditions"; and by doing so, it could, without resorting to regulation, promote an expanding economy and a "sounder," "more stable," more smoothly functioning one.[28] This was an idea that Hoover urged again and again during his first few months in office.[29]

Almost immediately, too, he set out to implement it, particularly by turning his Census Bureau into an agency that could provide "prophecy as well as history." In July, 1921, he launched the *Monthly Survey of Current Business*, which, by publishing census data on current industrial production and stocks, would serve as a guide for future decision-making in the private sector of the economy.[30] If such a publication had existed earlier, Hoover felt at the time, "the height of the last boom and the depth of the present slump could have been mitigated."[31] And in later years, he remained convinced that the service was a valuable one. It acted as "a counterpoise to 'psychology' in business—an anchor of basic facts [for businessmen] to tie to,"[32] and it had therefore contributed to the "remarkable period of stability" into which the country had entered.[33]

Hoover's acute awareness of "the larger role psychology played in the ebb and flow of business" also lay behind his publicity tactic of issuing press releases every New Year's Day discussing the "economic outlook" for the coming year. Carefully drafted to maintain "confidence" in the economy while pointing out potential dangers, the releases purveyed a tone of "cautious optimism" in their predictions of continuing prosperity. The secretary often made similar "confidence-building" statements on other occasions —most notably in the spring of 1926 when he felt the economy needed stabilizing following the collapse of the Florida real estate boom.[34]

Also essential to reconstruction and full employment, as Hoover saw it, was the restoration of foreign trade; and here, too, in his efforts to expand American commerce overseas, the compilation and dissemination of "fact information" played a vital role.[35] The idea was to gather, "sift out," and make trade intelligence "accessible to the business public"; and once the Bureau of Foreign and Domestic Commerce had been reorganized along commodity lines[36] and placed under the direction of Julius Klein, one of several men in Hoover's service "on loan" from Harvard University, the information did begin to flow. Especially significant in the dissemination of it was the daily *Commerce Report*, once "an insignificant pamphlet," but now transformed into a weekly magazine with carefully arranged trade data and "special articles of comment and counsel especially suited to the needs of business readers."[37] Also significant was the *Commerce Yearbook*, issued annually to summarize economic, commercial, and industrial developments throughout the world.[38] And along with these came hundreds of *Trade Information Bulletins*, presenting "timely and perishable" data for especially interested persons.[39]

In addition, there were special efforts to stimulate the interest of business and make it more aware of the information available. Klein, for example, insisted that his staff make the reports "really salable."[40] He arranged, as noted previously, for weekly pages of trade opportunities information in over 600 newspapers.[41] He affixed advertising "stickers" on all the bureau's outgoing correspondence, a practice, he reported, that had "a most favorable effect in increasing subscriptions."[42] And he kept the "press room on its toes to get out the most effective publicity" for the *Reports* and *Yearbooks.*[43] In all, he boasted to Hoover in October, 1925, the newspapers, during the preceding six months, had published "119,974 column inches" of the bureau's material, "more than enough to put eighteen columns of type set up and down the Washington Monument."[44]

As with the other Department of Commerce promotional activities, Hoover and Klein were also able to propagandize their foreign trade program in the business, trade, and popular press through their close working relationships with Arch Shaw of *System Magazine*, Frederick Feiker of McGraw Hill's trade journals, and Isaac Marcosson of the *Saturday Evening Post.* "As a result of publicity like this," a student of the secretary's "economic diplomacy" has written, "bills were presented to raise the budget of the Commerce Department and to safeguard its expanded functions by new legislation."[45] By facilitating the passage of favorable legislation as it advertised trade opportunities, his vigorous publicity effort, Hoover believed, had increased American sales abroad by "hundreds of millions of dollars annually."[46]

Also closely related to Hoover's "fact publicity" in the fields of foreign and domestic commerce was his public relations drive in support of the institution of the trade association. The trade association, as he saw it, was an ideal means for "holding in tandem" the conflicting yet indispensable social needs of "competition," the source of "individual initiative," and "cooperation," the producer of "economic stability."[47] It was an agency that should be encouraged and used by the government, one that was cooperating well in supplying the "production and distribution statistics" needed for "safer judgments" on business policy, aiding trade expansion and waste elimination, improving "business morals and practices," and promoting stable, yet unregulated, economic growth.[48] A tiny minority of such associations, to be sure, were in restraint of trade and "should be eliminated," but the "vast majority" were capable of "constructive cooperation";[49] and hence, it would be disastrous to accept the arguments being pushed by the Justice Department —the view, in other words, that all their activities "led to violations of the law" and that the antitrust laws should be stretched to prohibit them.[50]

To "reestablish confidence in the legitimate trade association," Hoover sought to clarify its legal status and marshal support behind it through a public relations campaign. He began with a press statement in 1921,[51] and then, following unfavorable court decisions, he addressed two letters to Attorney General Harry M. Daugherty—one in February, 1922, the second in December, 1923 —defending constructive associational activities and asking for legal clarification. In both instances, Daugherty's answers were guarded and not entirely satisfying. Yet Hoover felt that the juxtoposition of his inquiries with the attorney general's replies would be helpful, and he therefore released the exchanges for public scrutiny through his department's Press Bureau[52] and aired them in a *Commerce Report* and in *Outlook* magazine.[53] Following the initial letter, he also held a conference with trade association representatives, arranged for the publication of their statistics in areas conceded as legal by the attorney general, and secured national publicity for his conference address, a speech in which he advanced all his arguments in favor of the associations.[54] Later in the year, he reiterated his position in his widely publicized *Annual Report.*[55] Comparing the *Annual Reports of the Attorney General* of 1923 and 1924, Louis Galambos has concluded that "Hoover's defense of the associations gradually pushed the Justice Department to a new [more favorable] position."[56]

Frederick Feiker, whom Hoover had made chairman of a departmental committee dealing with trade associations, was meanwhile instrumental in mobilizing business opinion. Early in 1922, he secured arrangements whereby eleven of McGraw-Hill's trade journals printed commentary favorable to the "Chief's" position in his first exchange with Daugherty.[57] Later in the year, assisted by trade association representatives and members of the department's staff, he prepared a department publication entitled *Trade Association Activities*, the purpose of which, according to Hoover's introductory comment, was "to present a picture of the organization, administration, and operations of trade associations," both to "meet the need for public information on the subject" and to insure that "a business facility which is economically useful . . . may not suffer discrimination by reason of misapprehensions regarding its purposes and accomplishments."[58] To help it achieve these goals, the manual was given wide advance publicity in such magazines as the *Nation's Business* and *Printer's Ink* and in the house organs of such organizations as the Chamber of Commerce, the National Association of Manufacturers, the Associated Advertising Clubs of the World, the National Industrial Conference, and the American Automobile Association.[59] Advance orders alone, running as they did to 10,000 sales copies, were "far in excess of those received for any previous publication issued by the Department."[60]

Such publications and activities, moreover, did seem to influence both business and public opinion, and thus helped to save the cooperative machinery through which Hoover was working. In the opinion of the Department of Commerce solicitor, Stephen B. Davis, they provided "valuable aids and guides to legitimate associations."[61] And, as Hoover himself saw it, they succeeded in "causing much discussion" and having "important consequences," not the least of which was the sanctioning by the Supreme Court in 1925 of private statistical exchanges and related associational activities.[62]

Still another item of major importance in Hoover's program for "national reconstruction and development" was his multifaceted public relations campaign on behalf of housing reform and expansion. The need for increased home-building had been a theme of his addresses of the 1919-20 period. As a result of suspended construction during the war, he had estimated in 1920, "the country was short fully a million houses"; and if this shortage was to be overcome, the government did have a role to play, both in stimulating the building of homes and in expanding and rationalizing the construction industry. In this field, as in others, it should intervene "to induce active cooperation in the community itself."[63] Consequently, soon after assuming his duties as secretary of commerce, he asked for and received legislation creating a "Division of Building and Housing" in his department. This agency was in operation by June, 1921, and, under the direction of John M. Gries, it became another tool for "stimulating" cooperative action, an institution through and around which Hoover created publicity in the campaign for expanded housing.[64]

In doing so, moreover, he again followed his tested administrative pattern of "cooperation," "constructive study," and "ventilation of findings." After surveying community housing problems through conferences with municipal officials, engineers, and architects, he and Gries prepared a series of reports and "educational materials," which, if followed, could mitigate these problems and pave the way of a renewal of home construction.[65] Included were "model" plumbing and building codes, standard zoning regulations for cities, and general "common-sense information" for the prospective home-buyer.[66] Such reports, having been published by the Government Printing Office, were then "ventilated" to the public. Both Croghan and Lupton Wilkinson issued numerous press releases announcing the availability and contents of them, and before long, literally thousands of copies of the *Building Code Manual*, the *Zoning Primer*, and the *Own Your Own Home* booklet were being distributed.[67]

Large amounts of additional publicity also came from private organizations whose cooperation Hoover was able to solicit. The American Institute of Architects, for instance, broadcast the division's recommended building and plumbing codes through its press service of some twenty newspapers that, taken together, had a circulation of one and a half million subscribers.[68] The National Association of Real Estate Boards instructed its local boards to release the *Zoning Primer* and to secure publicity for it in the real

estate sections of their local newspapers.[69] And, of major importance, Hoover was able to take over and use the "Better Homes for
America" movement, founded by Mrs. William Brown Meloney,
editor of the women's magazine *Delineator*.

His association with the latter movement began in June, 1922,
when Donald Wilhelm, his publicity man in charge of magazines,
called his attention to the committees that Mrs. Meloney and the
Delineator were organizing in communities across the country and
urged him to extend full cooperation. "Strategically," both Wilhelm
and Gries "were agreed" that this campaign "was the best possible
opening for housing." It was "exactly the thing needed to shove
over the whole [*sic*] housing and better homes ideas of the Department."[70]

Hoover was quick to act on the recommendation. Within several days, he had sent a thousand copies of the *Zoning Primer* to
Mrs. Meloney, who promised to distribute them through her organization.[71] After consulting with her personally, he agreed to
join the "Advisory Council" of the Better Homes movement,[72] and
before long had become the organization's most prominent booster, assisting in its "Demonstration Home" exhibits and securing, in
his words, "advance blasts . . . of propaganda" for them by persuading the president to sign endorsements and by writing material for presidential speeches.[73] Once involved, moreover, he was
able to bring the movement under his control and to reorganize it
"in support of the Department's ideas."[74] In July, 1923, when the
publisher of the *Delineator*, G. W. Wilder, wrote that the management of the movement was becoming expensive and that he
could no longer sanction Mrs. Meloney's "personal direction and
promotion" of it,[75] Hoover proposed a new organization, in which
Wilder and Mrs. Meloney would be members of the executive
committee and the *Delineator* would continue its support, but fi-
nancing and management would come from other sources.
Wilder agreed, asking only that he be given recognition for "the
service rendered to America" by his initiation of the movement.[77]

Accordingly, in December, 1923, Hoover established a "public
service corporation" for housing, an organization in which he
would serve as president, Gries as treasurer,[78] and James Ford,

whom he had "borrowed" from Harvard University, as official director.[79] "In reality," as he himself put it, Better Homes in America was being transformed into "a sort of collateral arm to the Housing Division of the Department of Commerce";[80] and in successfully appealing to Col. Arthur Woods, a director of the Laura Spelman Foundation, for a three-year, $250,000 financial grant, he noted that "the competent staff under Dr. Gries in the Department of Commerce" would "provide continuously good administration." "Furthermore," he asserted, "on its propaganda side," he "would be able to assemble the men who have been associated with the American Relief Administration, that is, George Barr Baker, Frank Page, etc."[81]

In this new form, moreover, the Better Homes movement did provide Hoover with the machinery for a truly massive public relations campaign. By 1926, it had spawned more than 1,800 local committees, each celebrating "Better Homes Weeks," exhibiting "Demonstration Homes" in their communities,[82] and "ventilating" the "basic publicity" supplied by such Hoover aides as Lupton Wilkinson and Ray Mayer. These committees also undertook public relations campaigns of their own, mobilizing, in 1925, approximately $100,000 of regional newspaper and magazine publicity,[83] and reaching, through local demonstrations, lecture programs, and a film, "Home Sweet Home," supplied by the national office, an estimated three million people.[84] As a result, Hoover observed, the department's *Own Your Own Home* pamphlet was being sold by the "millions," and "years of experience and extensive research" were being "carried without waste motion to hundreds of thousands of families."[85]

Three years later, Hoover was even more satisfied with the results. By 1928, he claimed, 128 municipalities were using the department's building code recommendations, nearly 600 cities had adopted its model zoning ordinance, and the annual construction of dwelling units over the past six years had averaged 400,000 units higher than the figure for 1921.[86] All of this had helped to expand employment while meeting the "greatest social need of the country—more and better housing."[87] And just as important for Hoover, it had all been accomplished by methods that had avoided "direct government action" and had thus maintained "the free initiative of the people."[88]

The avoidance of "direct government action" and the maintenance of the "free initiative of the people" also figured prominently in the campaign that Hoover inaugurated early in his term as secretary of commerce against the rising tide of unemployment. Operating again from behind the scenes, he had opened this in August, 1921, by suggesting to Harding that he "appoint a Presidential Commission of men representative of all sections, predominantly those who can influence the action of employing forces and who can influence public opinion."[89] Harding, having acknowledged Hoover's "more intimate touch with the industrial and commercial situation" and having asked him to suggest men "who would make the conference a success,"[90] had then sent invitations to some one hundred leaders in business, labor, government, and academic life whom Hoover had recommended. And thus was born "The President's Conference on Unemployment," a conference that, in spite of its name, was directed by the secretary of commerce from start to finish.

With Hoover as its chairman and Edward Eyre Hunt, his administrative assistant, as its secretary, the conference, described by Christian Herter as "another one of those three ring affairs that the Chief likes to take on,"[91] assembled for three weeks in September and October, 1921. Addressing its opening session, Hoover set the tone for the proceedings by calling for "remedies outside the range of legislation," remedies which would avoid "that . . . paternalism" which would "undermine our whole political system." The role of the conference, as of government, he asserted, should be to "mobilize the intelligence of the country [so] that the . . . community [could] be instructed [in] the part [it could] play in effecting solutions."[92]

Accordingly, the conferees placed the primary "responsibility for leadership" upon the individual communities. Working through local emergency committees, they recommended, communities should expand public works, investigate means by which to facilitate the growth of private construction, and urge property owners, hotels, offices, and manufacturers to undertake "repairs, cleaning, and alterations" during the winter rather than in the spring.[93] To "stimulate," "assist," and "coordinate" these activities, there would be a central Committee on Civic and Emergency Measures to be chaired by Colonel Arthur Woods, who, as an assistant to the secretary of war, had recently been in charge of securing employment for former servicemen.[94] And finally, to "continue until the . . . unemployment emergency was passed," there would be a "standing committee," with Hoover remaining as chairman and Hunt as secretary. The latter agency would watch over the operations of the Woods committee, and, in addition, would undertake studies of the business cycle and construction industry with a view to discovering "permanent measures of preventing unemployment." To make these inquiries, it created two subcommittees, one chaired by Owen D. Young, president of the General Electric Company, the other by Ernest Trigg, a leading figure in the construction industry.[95]

If these studies and recommendations were to be implemented, however, the local communities and the public in general must understand them and be willing to cooperate. Hence, publicity became all-important, and to secure it, Hoover made full use of his department's publicity apparatus. His Press Bureau, for example, under Paul Croghan, dispatched numerous releases to the daily press. His old associate, Lupton A. Wilkinson, functioning now as "executive secretary in charge of publicity" for the conference, prepared many of these, describing, in particular, the preparations for the meeting, its aims, and the major resolutions and decisions it produced.[96] His assistant, E. E. Hunt, deeply concerned with "focusing public opinion on unemployment for the first time in American history," publicized the conference in speeches, magazine articles,[97] and a lengthy secretary's report distributed through the Commerce Department's Division of Publications.[98] Frederick Feiker persuaded the editors of McGraw-Hill's trade papers to disseminate the recommendations in both editorials and advertisements.[99] And Hoover himself appealed directly to such influential organizations as the Motion Picture Theatre Owners and the National Educational Association, urging them "to get back of every mayor" and to spread the "basic facts and proposals of the

Conference" in the "secondary schools and colleges of the country."[100] Concerned that "the Conference should have a chance to develop its ideas without being subject to attack" and "misrepresentation," he also carefully reviewed press accounts of the event and wrote rebuttals to editors who had been critical of it.[101]

While creating favorable attitudes, Hoover also sought to induce local action through the instrumentality of the Woods committee, which he headquartered in the Department of Commerce and "gave his personal direction."[102] For him, it became "a national clearing house of information"[103] functioning to "instruct the community," an agency that, in terms of his administrative theory, connected the "centralized ideas" of the conference to their "decentralized execution" in the communities. Having already addressed letters to all communities of more than 20,000 inhabitants,[104] and having secured "mayors' emergency committees" in 209 of the 327 cities solicited,[105] he and Woods then established a system of two-way communications, sending to the local committees the suggestions of the conference along with other literature on unemployment, receiving from them periodic "progress reports" as to what had been undertaken and accomplished, and using these reports to compile and dispatch bulletins that would enable the communities to benefit from shared experience.[106] Along with the bulletins, too, the committee sent field representatives to various sections of the country, where they explained to newspaper editors that they had come to inquire into the area's employment situation, and in this way, gave added impetus to efforts already being made on the local scene.[107]

Having insured that the recommendations of the President's Conference penetrated to the local communities, and having persuaded them to act, Hoover then sought to sustain national support through the generation of more publicity in the important news media of the country. Throughout the fall and winter of 1921 and 1922, his Press Bureau kept up a steady stream of releases, citing the methods, goals, and accomplishments of the national and local emergency committees. At the same time, Lupton Wilkinson and his assistants placed attention-getting copy with the leading magazines and newspapers of New York, San Francisco, and Washington, D.C.[108] When Wilkinson's contract with the Woods committee expired, his replacement, Major R. L. Foster, procured new reams of publicity, again by preparing and dispatching appropriate releases to news organs in every state of the Union. Especially well received was a little booklet of twenty-four editorials, featuring in particular local measures and achievements, the Hunt report, and the statements of Woods and Hoover. Designed "to keep before thinking persons the fact that there [was] still a situation to be faced,"[109] this booklet was sent to some 6,000 publications; and, as Foster later reported, "some newspapers printed every article . . . and many used two or three in a single day," generally, "on the editorial page."[110] The success of Foster's "one-man campaign," as he called it, was indicated by the "thousands of clippings" returned to him by the clipping service of the Department of Commerce.[111]

Both Hunt and Hoover were impressed. The former viewed the "great amount of editorial comment" as an essential contribution to the "strategy of the Woods committee."[112] And the latter believed that the publicity campaign had made it possible to carry out the "relief measures adopted by the President's Conference" and thus to overcome unemployment "in much less time than in any other depression in our history."[113] To fasten this firmly in the public mind, he emphasized the techniques that had been used and the results of them in his extensively publicized and disseminated *Annual Report* in 1922.[114]

Having stimulated emergency action, Hoover also continued his campaign for national education on the long-range unemployment problem. To further this and to discover "preventive measures," it will be recalled, two committees had been created: the Young committee, to investigate the relationship between unemployment and the business cycle, and the Trigg committee, to study employment patterns in the construction industry. For the former, Hoover had also secured the expertise of the National Bureau of Economic Research, plus a $50,000 grant from the Carnegie Foundation;[115] and once its research got under way in April, 1922, Hunt and Feiker prepared advance publicity for the forthcoming report *Business Cycles and Unemployment* and arranged for its publication by McGraw-Hill, a house always ready to extend full cooperation to the secretary of commerce.[116]

Once completed, too, the study was made the focus of national attention. The Commerce Department distributed some 3,500 copies of a pamphlet summarizing the findings and recommendations,[117] and Lupton Wilkinson, employing the devices used earlier by Major Foster, secured publicity in the magazines and mailed out over 10,000 "editorial booklets" to the newspapers.[118] Again Hoover was immensely pleased. He had "never known an economic investigation" that had received "anywhere near so much attention," he observed, as he looked over the "809 editorials and special articles" returned to his office by his clipping service.[119] Moreover, he was certain that the study's major recommendation, its advocacy of counter-cyclical public and private construction policies, had exerted a definite "effect on business policy." "By reason of the report" and the publicity given to it, he believed, "the peak of the dangerous upward swing" of the economy in the spring of 1923 had been "cut off."[120]

A month before the appearance of *Business Cycles and Unemployment,* Hoover had taken more direct measures to deflate the economy, yet, typically, his action took place behind the scenes and again involved the mobilization of newspaper publicity. On March 2, 1923, he wrote President Harding: "You are probably aware that the building trades are booming to an extent that has become dangerous. It is impossible for the Administration to throw out direct warnings without reactions that are in themselves dangerous. It is, however, desirable that we should do everything we can in the situation that might otherwise cause difficulty. . . ." Hoover's proposal was for Harding to address to him a note, "somewhat in the sense" of one that he was enclosing to the president, asking for advice on government construction policy. Hoover would then make a "constructive reply showing the volume of construction going on and recommending that public work[s] be retarded. . . ." Harding assented to this stratagem, and Hoover then published their "exchange" of correspondence in a Department of Commerce press release. Printed in the New York *Times*, the release served to communicate Hoover's warning.[121]

Meanwhile, the Trigg committee was pursuing its studies; and just as in the case of the business cycle report, its findings, *Seasonal Operation in the Construction Industries*, were given advanced publicity by Hunt and Feiker and, when they appeared in July, 1924, were nationally publicized through the Department of Commerce Press Bureau and the professional work of Wilkinson.[122] Containing a foreword by the secretary himself, the study generally reinforced the findings of the Young committee, especially by recognizing the construction industry as the "balance wheel of the economy" and recommending a lengthening of the building season to eliminate seasonal idleness.[123] And again, the "cooperative activities established in the 'follow-up'" were felt by Hoover "to have had a marked effect" in "extending the building season into the winter months" and thus stabilizing employment.[124]

While using this public relations approach to control the fluctuations of the business cycle and promote steady economic expansion, Hoover had also become involved in another major campaign, one that better than any of the others, perhaps, reveals the studied manner in which he mobilized newspaper publicity in the service of his political philosophy. This was his behind-the-scenes struggle to abolish the twelve-hour day and eighty-four-hour week that persisted in a sizeable section of the steel industry. Believing that "commerce and industry could make [no] progress unless labor advanced with them," he began, in early 1922, by having his department prepare a study of the steel industry, the results of which indicated that the working hours were not only "barbaric" but "uneconomic" as well. "With the facts in hand" and with the approval of Secretary of Labor James J. Davis, he then induced President Harding, in April, 1922, to invite the steel manufacturers to a White House dinner conference.[125] He also suggested "making some public announcement of the purpose of the meeting before . . . it assembled," thus guaranteeing a "favorable impression in the country" and, more importantly, placing "a certain moral pressure on these gentlemen to take action. . . ."[126] When it came to making such a "flourish from the White House," however, Harding "hesitated"; and perhaps as a result, the unpublicized conference became an "acrid debate" between Hoover and the steel magnates, one that ended inconclusively with the industry's leaders promising to "investigate" themselves through a committee chaired by Judge Elbert H. Gary.[127]

Much "disheartened," "in less than good humor," and fearful that through intransigence the industry might find itself "smashed by some kind of legislation," the secretary turned next to his ancient strategy, that of "laying the matter before the public."[128] Emerging from the conference, he "startled" the representatives of the press by divulging that the president was trying to persuade the steel men to shorten the hours of their workers by one-third, thus provoking a "great public discussion" and, according to his estimates, placing "ninety per cent of the public opinion of the entire country . . . solidly behind the President."[129] Then, when the industry still failed to move, he instigated the preparation of another report, this time by a committee of the Federated American Engineering Societies, a body, as noted previously, that he had presided over in 1920-21. Completed on November 1, 1922, the report strongly recommended the adoption of the eight-hour day; and to enhance the impact of the volume, Hoover persuaded Harding to sign a foreword in which he eulogized the findings as being in the best "interests of good citizenship, of business, and of economic stability."[130]

In spite of the presidential endorsement, though, and in spite of the fact that the secretary "kept the pot boiling in the press,"[131] it was not until July, 1923, that such pressure tactics finally bore fruit. Reporting in May, Judge Gary's committee had promised little action and, for Hoover, had displayed a distressing "inability to grasp the great ground swell of social movements amongst our people." Determined that "this matter of fundamental social concern" should not be dropped, Hoover had reacted by drafting a letter for the president to send to Gary, one that had expressed great disappointment in the report and suggested a change from two to three shifts as a means of shortening working hours. "Such an undertaking," it had concluded, "would give great satisfaction to the American people . . . and . . . establish confidence in the ability of our industries to solve themselves matters so conclusively advocated by the public."[132] Given great publicity, the letter had alarmed Gary, and the latter, with the concurrence of the directors of the American Iron and Steel Institute, had finally notified the president that steps were being taken for the "total abolition of the twelve-hour day."[133] To seal the triumph, Hoover had the exchange of correspondence released to the press and persuaded the president to make the news of Gary's retreat the major part of one of his last speeches, that delivered in Tacoma, Washington, on July 5, 1923.[134] True to the guidelines he had established previously, Hoover had brought a measure of economic justice to the steel industry, not with "legal repression," but through the "organized pressure of public opinion."[135]

Hoover's campaigns for waste elimination, for "fact information" and associational activities, for housing, employment, and the "eight-hour day" were central to his quest for "national reconstruction and development," and in each of them, he utilized publicity as a major administrative tool. He also employed similar tactics, though on a smaller scale, in a multitude of other areas, in the development, for example, of the nation's water and power resources, the efficient operation of the coal and railroad industries, the conservation of fish, the control of water and air pollution, the development and regulation of the radio and aviation industries, and the creation of automobile traffic safety standards. By means of his Commerce Department public relations apparatus and with the assistance of his many influential friends in the daily and periodical press, he brought the "organized pressure of public opinion" to bear on all these matters; and in each case, with the exception of the coal problem, he believed that this had produced effective reforms, which in turn had contributed to economic growth and the spread of social stability.[136]

Just as important for him, however, was the political concomitant of his public relations approach, the notion that his uses of publicity, of conferences, and of cooperating committees were "perhaps the first steps in a new conception of government," one that would move away from centralized authority and rely upon "stimulation of the local community to its responsibilities and the education of the local community to intelligent action." This, he felt, was "a far wiser [method of governing] than the constant drive to centralize the government of the United States."[137] And campaigning for this "American system," as he labeled it in 1928,[138] he was able to capitalize on his renown and his innumerable ties with the mass media and win the presidential election by a landslide. Yet, as we shall see, against the background of economic depression, Hoover's public relations style, once so productive for the nation and, though largely unwittingly, for his own political fortune, would suddenly become a tremendous liability. A difficult period for even the most skillful of political leaders, the years 1929-33 would be years of unmitigated disaster for a man of Hoover's administrative approach, personality, and philosophy.

1. In response to a letter from Franklin Lane who had expressed concern that Hoover might not "find political life possible," Hoover acknowledged: "I am indeed greatly touched by your note and I feel everything you say. I pursued every alley in endeavor to find an excuse for refusing this position and each one of them became a blind alley to my own conscience. I realize that the surrounding forces in and out of the government are such that any one man can do but little. In these times I doubt whether any man has the right to refuse to take service lest he could accuse himself of something that he could have at least partially mitigated. I do recognize that I am not intellectually constituted for this kind of job and that bold diagnosis and strong action are not consonant with our political institution[s] except in times of emergency." Franklin Lane to Hoover, March 1, 1921; Hoover to Lane, March 8, 1921, Secretary of Commerce Personal File, "Lane, Franklin," HHP, HHPL.

2. The sentence from the enabling act that struck Hoover's eye was: "It shall be the province and duty of the said Department to foster, promote, and develop the foreign and domestic commerce, the mining, manufacturing, shipping and fishery industries, the labor interests and the transportation facilities of the United States" (Herbert Hoover, *The Memoirs of Herbert Hoover, 1920-1933: The Cabinet and the Presidency*, 2:40).

3. Ibid., p. 36.

4. Secretary of Commerce Official File, "Press Releases, 1921-1928," HHP, HHPL.

5. "Press Release on the Department of Commerce," March 11, 1921, 134, Public Statements, HHP, HHPL.

6. Herbert Hoover, *Annual Report of the Secretary of Commerce* (Washington, 1925), p. 2.

7. Ibid.

8. Herbert Hoover, *Annual Report of the Secretary of Commerce* (Washington, 1924), p. 10.

9. Arch Shaw to Hoover, November 23, 1922, SCOF, "Shaw, A. W., 1921-1922," HHP, HHPL.

10. Bernard M. Baruch to Hoover, April 27, 1921, SCOF, "Baruch, Bernard," HHP, HHPL.

11. Hoover, Address before the American Engineering Councils Executive Board, February 14, 1921, 128, Public Statements, HHP, HHPL.

12. Edward E. Hunt, ed., *Waste in Industry*. Hoover wrote a foreword to the volume summarizing the findings.

13. Draft of article "Simplification" prepared by R. M. Hudson for the September, 1924, meeting of the National Conference of Business Paper Editors, SCOF, "National Conference of Business Paper Editors, 1924," HHP, HHPL.

14. Ibid.

15. Christian Herter to Albert W. Atwood, January 29, 1922; Donald Wilhelm to Herter, February 6, 1922, SCOF, "Commerce, Standards, Bureau of, Wilhelm, Donald," HHP, HHPL; Wilhelm, "Mr. Hoover as Secretary of Commerce"; Frederick Feiker, Speech before the National Editorial Conference, October 25, 1921; Feiker, "What the Commerce Department Is Doing for Industry," pp. 71-73; Feiker, "The Trend of 'Simplification': How the Movement Is Growing and What the Paving Brick Action Signifies," pp. 156-58; Feiker, "The Profession of Commerce in the Making." A member of the Planning Committee of the Division of Simplified Practice, Arch Shaw promoted the division's work in speeches and articles: Shaw, "Startling Statements," p. 534; Shaw, Speech before the Reunion of the War Industries Board, November, 1922; Shaw, "Simplification: A Philosophy of Business Management," pp. 417-27. See also the articles on simplification in the January, 1925, issue of *Factory*. SCOF, "Shaw, A. W.," HHP, HHPL. "As a backing to [his] campaign on simplification," Hoover had Shaw prepare a small book on the subject which was published as a "public document" by the department (Hoover to Shaw, March 12, 1923; Shaw to Hoover, June 13, 1923, SCOF, "Shaw, A.W.," HHP, HHPL).

16. R. C. Mayer to G. B. Baker, September 22, 1923, American Child Health Association, "Baker, G.B.," HHP, HHPL; Memorandum, Ernest L. Priest to Hudson, "Publicity for Simplified Practice during Period February 1, 1924,—January 1, 1925," SCOF, "Commerce, Simplified Commercial Practice, 1924-28," HHP, HHPL; Priest, "What Can Simplified Practice Do for the Restaurant Industry?", *Restaurant Man*, August, 1926.

17. Hoover to Samuel Insull, president of Commonwealth Edison Co., from whom he had "borrowed" Durgin, March 2, 1923; "Report of Division of Simplified Practice Planning Committee Meeting," November 22, 1923, SCOF, "Commerce, Simplified Commercial Practice, 1921-22," HHP, HHPL.

18. Hoover to S. W. Stratton, director of Bureau of Standards, February 15, 1922; Bulletin, "Simplified Practice: What It Is and What It Offers," July 21, 1922, SCOF, "Commerce, Simplified Commercial Practice, 1921-22"; Hudson to Hoover, "Quarterly Report on Activities of the Division of Simplified Practice," August 13, 1924, SCOF, "Commerce, Simplified Commercial Practice, 1924-28," HHP, HHPL.

19. Draft of article "Simplification" prepared by Hudson for National Conference of Business Paper Editors, SCOF, "National Conference of Business Paper Editors, 1924," HHP, HHPL.

20. Department of Commerce Press Release, "Find Simplified Practice New Source of Gain," August 13, 1924, SCOF, "Commerce, Simplified Commercial Practice, 1924-1928," HHP, HHPL.

21. Hoover, *Annual Report of the Secretary of Commerce*, 1925, pp. 2-29; *Annual Report of the Secretary of Commerce* (Washington, 1926), pp. 2-28.

22. Memorandum, Hudson to Hoover, "Progress in Simplified Practice," July 15, 1927, SCOF, "Commerce, Simplified Commercial Practice, 1924-1928," HHP, HHPL.

23. Department of Commerce Press Release, "Find Simplified Practice New Source of Gain"; *Annual Reports*, 1925, 1926.

24. Hoover, "Remarks at the Brick Makers' Conference," November 15, 1921, 185B, Public Statements, HHP, HHPL. The effectiveness of Hoover's simplification publicity in penetrating the national consciousness may be suggested by the fact that from the perspective of several social historians writing in the 1930s, the secretary's simplification work was his most noteworthy achievement (Mark Sullivan, *Our Times: The Twenties*, 6:648-49; Preston W. Slosson, *The Great Crusade and After, 1914-1928*, pp. 186-87.

25. Milton N. Nelson, "The Effect of Open Price Association Activities," *American Economic Review* 13 (June, 1923): 258-75.

26. Hoover, *Memoirs*, 2:75.

27. Hoover to Howard Sutherland, senator from West Virginia, May 14, 1921, SCOF, "Senate," Hoover Papers; Hoover, *Annual Report of the Secretary of Commerce* (Washington, 1921), p. 6.

28. Hoover, "Fact Information in Business," *Special Libraries*, April, 1921, 140B, Public Statements, HHP, HHPL.

29. Ibid.; Hoover, Address at the New York *Commercial's* One Hundred and Twenty-Fifth Anniversary, May 23, 1921, 157, Public Statements, HHP, HHPL (published in New York *Commercial* and distributed in leaflets by the American Exchange National Bank); Hoover, Commerce Department Press Release, "The Federal Trade Commission Law," 158, Public Statements, HHP, HHPL (published in New York *Times*, June 3, 1921).

30. Hoover, *Memoirs*, 2:176; Feiker, "What the Department of Commerce Is Doing for Industry," p. 73; Wilhelm, "Mr. Hoover As Secretary of Commerce," pp. 409-10.

31. Hoover, Address at the New York *Commercial's* One Hundred and Twenty-Fifth Anniversary.

32. Hoover, Address before the National Distribution Conference of the Chambers of Commerce of the United States, January 14, 1925, 435, Public Statements, HHP, HHPL (published in *Nation's Business*, March, 1925); Commerce Department Press Release, "Figures [of *Survey of Current Business*] Show Improvement in January," February 12, 1922, SCOF, "Press Release," HHP, HHPL.

33. Hoover to David Lawrence, editor of the *United States Daily*, December 29, 1927, 811, Public Statements, HHP, HHPL (published in the *United States Daily*, January 3, 1928).

34. Hoover, "New Year's Day Statements," Public Statements, 195, 277, 342, 428, 537, 689, 814, HHP, HHPL; Hoover, "Prosperity Will March On," March 5, 1926, 559B, Public Statements, HHP, HHPL (published in New York *Times*, New York *Herald Tribune*, and *Commercial and Financial Chronicle*); Hoover, "Avoid Reckless Speculation and Prosperity Will Continue," Staunton *News-Leader*, March 21, 1926, 563, Public Statements, HHP, HHPL; Hoover to Arthur Robinson, editor of *Collier's Magazine*, April 22, 1926, SCPF, HHP, HHPL; "Statement by Secretary Hoover Given to Isaac Marcosson for the *Saturday Evening Post*," June 22, 1926, SCPF, HHP, HHPL.

35. Hoover, *Memoirs* 2:79.

36. The section of the staff of the Bureau of Foreign and Domestic Commerce working overseas to send "trade intelligence" back to the department had formerly been organized on a geographic basis. Hoover's reorganization was to deploy these men on a commodity basis. The bureau's agents, in other words, no longer reported their "trade opportunities" to a European or South American "division" but reported them directly to the appropriate industry. In this way, trade intelligence could be efficiently filtered through the trade associations (Feiker, "What the Department of Commerce Is Doing for Industry," pp. 71-73; Wilhelm, "Mr. Hoover As Secretary of Commerce," pp. 407-10).

37. Draft of article "Bureau of Foreign and Domestic Commerce" prepared by Julius Klein for the September, 1924, meeting of the National Conference of Business Paper Editors, SCOF, "National Conference of Business Paper Editors, 1924," HHP, HHPL.

38. Ibid.

39. Ibid.

40. Hoover, *Memoirs*, 2:79; Klein to Hoover, April 24, 1925, SCOF, "Commerce, Publicity," HHP, HHPL.

41. Klein, Draft of article for the National Conference of Business Paper Editors.

42. Klein to Hoover, April 24, 1925, SCOF, "Commerce, Publicity," HHP, HHPL.

43. Ibid. As a result, the bureau was able to increase the number of *Yearbooks* it distributed from 3,200 in 1922 to 8,100 in 1923. Klein expected to sell 15,000 copies of the 1924 edition of the *Yearbook*.

44. Klein to Hoover, April 16, 1925; Klein to Hoover, October 15, 1925, SCOF, "Commerce, Publicity," HHP, HHPL.

45. Joseph Brandes, *Herbert Hoover and Economic Diplomacy: Department of Commerce Policy, 1921-1928*, p. 57. Brandes' study offers a detailed description of Hoover's use of public relations to expand trade. See, especially, pages 10-21. Hoover's related publicity campaign via "press releases, pamphlets, and fervent addresses" to protect American manufacturing and consumer interests against "monopolistic" foreign exporters, Brandes feels, was also successful in securing appropriations "enabling the Commerce Department to conduct a world-wide search for independent supplies of raw materials under United States control" (pp. 215-16).

46. Hoover, *Memoirs*, 2:79.

47. Feiker, "What the Department of Commerce Is Doing for Industry," pp. 71-73; Hoover to Edwin F. Cay, Editor of New York *Evening Post*, March 15, 1922, SCOF, "Press Releases," HHP, HHPL.

48. Ibid.

49. Ibid.

50. Hoover, *Memoirs*, 2:169.

51. Hoover, Department of Commerce Press Release, "Federal Trade Commission Law," June 2, 1921, 158, Public Statements, HHP, HHPL (published in New York *Times*, June 3, 1921).

52. Hoover, Department of Commerce Press Releases, "Trade Association Activities—Correspondence," February 16, 1922 and January 10, 1924, SCOF, "Press Releases," HHP, HHPL.

53. *Commerce Reports*, February 20, 1922; Hunt, "Government and Trade Associations."

54. Hoover, Department of Commerce Press Releases, March 17, 1922 and April 12, 1922, SCOF, "Press Releases," HHP, HHPL.

55. Hoover, *Annual Report of the Secretary of Commerce*, 1921; Department of Commerce Press Release, "The Restraint of Trade Acts" (from *Annual Report*), December 2, 1922, SCOF, "Press Releases," HHP, HHPL.

56. Louis Galambos, *Competition and Cooperation: The Emergence of a National Trade Association*, p. 94.

57. Feiker to Herter, February 28, 1922, SCOF, "Feiker, F.M., 1921-1922," HHP, HHPL.

58. Memorandum, "Secretary Hoover's Book on Trade Associations," December 8, 1922, SCOF, "Trade Associations, Trade Associations' Activities," HHP, HHPL; Hoover, "Trade Association Activities," July 15, 1923, 319 Public Statements, HHP, HHPL.

59. Memorandum, "Trade Association Activities," July 11, 1923, SCOF, "Trade Associations, Trade Associations' Activities," HHP, HHPL.

60. T. F. McKeon to Hoover, June 15, 1923, SCOF, "Trade Associations, Trade Associations' Activities," HHP, HHPL.

61. Draft of article "Trade Associations" prepared by Stephen B. Davis for the September, 1924, meeting of the National Conference of Business Paper Editors, SCOF, "National Conference of Business Paper Editors, 1924," HHP, HHPL.

62. *Memoirs*, 2:170. With the legal battle won, Hoover continued to promote the cause of the trade association in speeches and articles. The institution remained for him a key to that "great transformation" that he perceived in the political economy of the country and that he desired to aid and abet: the transformation of regulated "extreme individualism" into unregulated "associational activities" (Hoover, "The Limits of Responsibilities of Legislation as Related to Business," Address before the California State Business Committee, November 7, 1924, 410A, Public Statements, HHP, HHPL).

63. Herbert Hoover, "The Housing Problem: A Direct Message for Responsible Industrial Executives," 106, Public Statements, HHP, HHPL.

64. Memorandum enclosing draft of bill establishing the Division of Building and Housing, F. T. Miller to Hoover, April 22, 1921, SCOF, "Building and Housing, Miller, F. T., 1921," HHP, HHPL; Hoover to Warren G. Harding, February 9, 1922, SCOF, "Unemployment, Harding, President Warren G.," HHP, HHPL.

65. Draft of article "Building and Housing" prepared by John M. Gries for the September, 1924, meeting of the National Conference of Business Paper Editors, SCOF, "National Conference of Business Paper Editors, 1924," HHP, HHPL.

66. Ibid.; Hoover, "America A Nation of Homes Is the Goal of Many Forces," *Christian Science Monitor*, March 25, 1925, 460, Public Statements, HHP, HHPL.

67. Gries to Hoover, July 6, 1922; Gries to Hoover, August 3, 1922; Press Release, "Standard Zoning Law," September 15, 1922, SCOF, "Building and Housing—Zoning"; Press Release, "Own Your Own Home," September 9, 1923; William Mullendore, assistant to Hoover, to Wilkinson, September 17, 1923; R. C. Mayer, vice-president of Lupton Wilkinson, Inc., to Christian Herter, November 16, 1923, SCOF, "Building and Housing"; Herter to Mayer, October 5, 1923; Press Clippings, September 28, 1923, SCPF, "Mayer, R.C."; Press Release, "Jumbled Cities," July 3, 1922; Press Release, "Conferences on Housing," December 1, 1922; Press Re-

lease, "Zoning Progress," January 29, 1923; Mullendore to Wilkinson, September 1, 1923, SCOF, "Building and Housing," HHP, HHPL.

68.   Gries to Hoover, May 1, 1922; clipping from *World's Work* (April, 1922), SCOF, "Building and Housing," HHP, HHPL.

69.   The Publicity Department of the National Association of Real Estate Boards regarded its "Zoning Primer" material for the press as "by far the most important ever released" by the organization. All local boards were instructed "to handle it with great care" (Don D. Goss to Secretaries of All Boards, May 8, 1922, SCOF, "Building and Housing," HHP, HHPL). Gries noted to Hoover that "as you pointed out last year, many of the people we are most anxious to reach are likely to see articles in the real estate sections of newspapers." In planning the Division's press releases, he was "keeping that fact in mind" (Gries to Hoover, February 13, 1923, SCOF, "Building and Housing," HHP, HHPL).

70.   Donald Wilhelm to Hoover, June 22, 1922, SCOF, "Commerce, Standards, Bureau of, Wilhelm, Donald," HHP, HHPL.

71.   Mrs. William Brown Meloney to G. B. Baker, June 26, 1922, George Barr Baker Papers, Box 5, Hoover Institution on War, Revolution, and Peace.

72.   Hoover to George B. Christian, Jr., secretary to President Harding, August 29, 1922, SCOF, "Meloney, Mrs. William Brown," HHP, HHPL.

73.   Ibid.; Herbert Hoover, "The Home as An Investment," 260, Public Statements, HHP, HHPL; Hoover, "Better Homes Campaign"—Letter to J. A. Hunter, New Haven Chamber of Commerce, 274A, Public Statements, HHP, HHPL (published in New Haven *Union*, January 4, 1923, and the *Delineator*, May, 1923); Hoover to Harding, February 2, 1923; Hoover to Harding, June 1, 1923, SCOF, "Building and Housing—Better Homes in America," HHP, HHPL.

74.   Hoover, *Memoirs*, 2:93.

75.   G. W. Wilder to Hoover, July 20, 1923, SCOF, "Building and Housing —Better Homes in America," HHP, HHPL.

76.   Hoover to Wilder, October 4, 1923, SCOF, "Building and Housing—Better Homes in America," HHP, HHPL.

77.   Mrs. Meloney to Hoover, December 15, 1923; Wilder to Hoover, December 31, 1923, SCOF, "Building and Housing—Better Homes in America," HHP, HHPL. Mrs. Meloney did remain with Better Homes as an executive director, and the *Delineator* remained an important forum for Hoover's ideas on housing, child health, and other issues as well.

78.   Mrs. Meloney to Hoover, December 15, 1923; Herter to Philip Welch, December 21, 1923, SCOF, "Building and Housing—Better Homes in America," HHP, HHPL.

79.   Hoover, *Memoirs*, 2:92; Hoover to A. Lawrence Lowell, December 28, 1923, SCOF, "Lowell, Dr. A. Lawrence," Hoover Papers. Hoover had become a close friend of the president of Harvard University, A. Lawrence Lowell, during the war years and had assisted Lowell's efforts to induce Republican party leaders to support the League of Nations in 1920. As secretary of commerce, he called upon Lowell on several occasions "to discommode yourself and your students" by granting leaves of absence to faculty members for "government service" (Hoover to Lowell, September 23, 1927, SCOF, "Lowell, Dr. A. Lawrence," HHP, HHPL).

80.   Hoover thus described the new Better Homes organization in a letter to President Coolidge asking for an endorsement of the movement (Hoover to Calvin Coolidge, January 9, 1924, SCOF, "Building and Housing—Better Homes in America," HHP, HHPL).

81. Hoover to Woods, November 21, 1923, SCOF, "Building and Housing—Better Homes in America"; Hoover to Lowell, December 28, 1923, SCOF, "Lowell, Dr. A. Lawrence," HHP, HHPL.

82. Memorandum, James Ford to Mrs. Meloney, January 14, 1926, SCOF, "Building and Housing—Better Homes in America," HHP, HHPL.

83. Ibid.; Wilkinson to George Akerson, January 31, 1927, SCOF, "Building and Housing—Better Homes in America," HHP, HHPL.

84. James Ford to Mrs. Meloney, January 14, 1926, SCOF, "Building and Housing—Better Homes in America," HHP, HHPL.

85. *Memoirs*, 2:93; Herbert Hoover, "America A Nation of Homes Is the Goal of Many Forces," *Christian Science Monitor*.

86. *Memoirs*, 2:94-96.

87. Ibid.

88. Hoover, "America A Nation of Homes." It should be noted here that Hoover mobilized a massive public relations campaign, very similar in technique and purpose to his housing effort, in the field of child health. As president of the Child Health Association, he desired to "put health over as a national theme," and therefore directed the ARA publicity staff, under George Barr Baker, and the staff of Lupton A. Wilkinson, Inc., to publicize the manifold activities and publications of the association. Among "the millions of these publications issued to "inspire the public" was Hoover's own "Child's Bill of Rights," which was published extensively. Although not directly related to the welfare of the economy, the child health drive was viewed by Hoover as a means of achieving long-term social stability without the imposition of federal controls. A frequently used refrain in his articles and speeches on the issue ran as follows: "If we could grapple with the whole child situation for one generation, our public health, our economic efficiency, the moral character, sanity and stability of our people would advance three generations in one. These complex problems cannot be solved by any iron-clad system of governmental action. . . . [But] much can be done by the waking of public conscience in every community." Hoover, Address before the American Child Hygiene Association, October 11, 1920, 93, Public Statements, HHP, HHPL; Index to Vol. 12 of Public Statements, "Bill of Rights," February, 1923, HHP, HHPL; Hoover, "A Little Child Shall Lead," *Good Housekeeping*, June, 1923, 312, Public Statements, HHP, HHPL; Hoover to Baker, October 31, 1922, SCOF, HHP, HHPL; Baker, Office Memorandum, "The American Child Health Association and the A.R.A.," February, 1923, ACHA, "Baker, G.B."; R. C. Mayer, "Report of the Publicity Department [of the] American Child Health Association," March 28, 1923, ACHA, "Publicity," HHP, HHPL; Hoover, *Memoirs*, 2:97-100.

89. Hoover to Harding, August 20, 1921, SCOF, "Unemployment, President," HHP, HHPL.

90. Harding to Hoover, August 24, 1921, SCOF, "Unemployment, President," HHP, HHPL.

91. Herter to Hugh Gibson, October 5, 1921, Hugh Gibson Collection, Box 7A, Hoover Institution on War, Revolution, and Peace.

92. Hoover, "National Unemployment Conference Address," September 26, 1921, 175, Public Statements, HHP, HHPL.

93. Edward Eyre Hunt, ed., *Report of the President's Conference on Unemployment*, pp. 19-21.

94. Ibid., pp. 17-18.

95. Ibid., pp. 18-19.

96. Ibid., p. 14; Commerce Department Press Releases September 20, September 26, October 4, October 10, October 12, and October 13, 1921, SCOF, "Press Releases," Hoover Papers; Lupton A. Wilkinson to Hunt, October 3, 1921, SCOF, "Unemployment, Wilkinson, Lupton A.," HHP, HHPL.

97. Hunt, "A Long Step Forward," pp. 427-29.

98. Hunt, *Report of the President's Conference on Unemployment*; T. F. Mc-Keon, director of Division of Publications, to Hunt, April 11, 1922, SCOF, "Unemployment, McKeon, Mr. T. F.," HHP, HHPL.

99. Feiker to A. A. Clifford, October 8, 1921, SCOF, "Unemployment, Mc-Graw-Hill Book Company," HHP, HHPL.

100. Hoover to Motion Picture Theater Owners, October 3, 1921, SCOF, "Unemployment, Hoover, Secretary"; Hoover to J. W. Crabtree, secretary of the National Education Association, September 30, 1921, SCOF, "Unemployment, National Educational Association," HHP, HHPL.

101. Hoover to Charles M. Lincoln, editor of the New York *Herald*, October 6, 1921; Hoover to the Editors of the *Journal of Commerce*, October 6, 1921; Hoover to Henry H. Lewis, editor of *Industry*, October 8, 1921, SCOF, "Unemployment, Periodicals," HHP, HHPL.

102. Hoover, *Memoirs*, 2:46.

103. Hunt, *Report of the President's Conference*, p. 171.

104. Hoover to all state governors, October 11, 1921, SCOF, "Unemployment, Governors, Communications to," HHP, HHPL.

105. Hunt, *Report of the President's Conference*, p. 172.

106. For examples of magazine articles on unemployment sent to the mayors, see Arthur Woods to Lupton Wilkinson, October 10, 1921, SCOF, "Unemployment, Magazines," and Woods to Hartford Powel, Jr., editor of *Collier's Weekly*, December 17, 1921, SCOF, "Unemployment, Publicity," HHP, HHPL. For the use of the "progress reports" and "bulletins," see Woods to Ben D. Brickhouse, mayor of Little Rock, Arkansas, October 13, 1921, and Woods to all mayors, March 17, 1922, SCOF, "Unemployment, Municipal," HHP, HHPL.

107. Transcript of minutes of meeting between Woods and field representatives, December 23, 1921; Department of Commerce Press Release "The President's Conference Is Sending Men to Selected Localities to Ascertain the Situation," December, 1921, SCOF, "Unemployment, Herrick, Mr. S. A.," HHP, HHPL.

108. Wilkinson to Woods, October 14, 1921; Wilkinson to Woods, October 15, 1921; Wilkinson to Woods, October 18, 1921, SCOF, "Unemployment, Publicity," HHP, HHPL.

109. Woods's preface to the "Editorial Booklet," March 6, 1922, SCOF, "Unemployment, Publicity," HHP, HHPL.

110. The editorials bore such titles as "Hoover on Unemployment," "Keeping them on the Payrolls," "Ten Helps for Slack Periods," "A Tale of Ten Cities," and the "Evils of Seasonal Unemployment." SCOF, "Editorial Booklet," March 6, 1922; Memorandum, Foster to Hunt, May 8, 1922, SCOF, "Unemployment, Publicity," and "Unemployment, Publicity Report," HHP, HHPL.

111. Memorandum, Foster to Hunt, May 8, 1922, SCOF, "Unemployment, Publicity Report," HHP, HHPL.

112. Memorandum, Hunt to Foster, March 28, 1922, SCOF, "Unemployment, Foster, Col. R. L.,"; Hunt to Wilkinson, April 29, 1922, SCOF, "Unemployment, Wilkinson, Lupton A.," HHP, HHPL.

113. Hoover, *Annual Report of the Secretary of Commerce*, 1924, p. 11.

114. Hoover, *Annual Report of the Secretary of Commerce* (Washington, 1922), pp. 6-7.

115. Edwin F. Gay to Hoover, October 22, 1921; Hunt to Henry S. Pritchett, president of the Carnegie Corporation of New York, December 29, 1921; Transcript of minutes of the "Business Cycle Meeting" held at Department of Commerce, April 13, 1922, SCOF, "Unemployment, National Bureau of Economic Research," HHP, HHPL.

116. As part of an "educational movement" to give the "businessman an intelligent understanding . . . of the business cycle," Feiker arranged for Hunt to prepare an article in *Printer's Ink* on the work of the committee. Entitled "How Industry Can Avoid Summer Depression," the article appeared in the magazine on May 18, 1922. Feiker to Hunt, May 4, 1922, SCOF, "Unemployment, Feiker, F. M."; Memorandum, Hunt to Emmet, May 9, 1922, SCOF, "Unemployment, Hunt, E. E."; Hunt to Feiker, July 6, 1922, SCOF, "Unemployment, Feiker, F. M." Even before the committee had actually assembled, Hoover had begun to build interest in the business cycle study through department press releases. "To Study Basic Causes of Unemployment," SCOF, "Press Releases"; also, Foster's release, March 9, 1922, SCOF, "Unemployment, Foster, Colonel R. L.," HHP, HHPL.

117. Hunt to Wilkinson, February 23, 1923; Memorandum to T. F. McKeon, April 20, 1923, SCOF, "Unemployment, Wilkinson, Lupton A.," HHP, HHPL.

118. Hunt to Wilkinson, March 20, 1923; Wilkinson to Hunt, May 16, 1923, SCOF, "Unemployment, Wilkinson, Lupton A.," HHP, HHPL. Newspaper articles taken from the booklet were sent to the department by its clipping service, Henry Romeike. The hundreds of clippings are filed in SCOF, "Unemployment, Publicity," HHP, HHPL. The report was also announced by a Department of Commerce press release of April 2, 1923, SCOF, "Unemployment, Wilkinson, Lupton A.," HHP, HHPL.

119. Ray Mayer, vice-president Lupton A. Wilkinson, Inc., to Hunt, February 23, 1923, SCOF, "Unemployment, Wilkinson, Lupton A.," HHP, HHPL. Hoover's enthusiasm for the publicity given the report is expressed in a letter he drafted to be sent to Elihu Root, chairman of the board of the Carnegie Corporation. Though for some reason it was never mailed, the letter well documents Hoover's belief in the efficacy of publicity in shaping economic policy in the private sector of the economy (Unsent letter, Hoover to Root, October 9, 1923, SCPF, HHP, HHPL).

120. Ibid.; also *Annual Report of the Secretary of Commerce*, 1924, p. 11.

121. Hoover to Harding, March 2, 1923, SCOF, "Construction, 1923"; Department of Commerce Press Release, March 17, 1923, SCOF, "Press Releases," HHP, HHPL; New York *Times*, March 19, 1923.

122. Commerce Department Press Release, July 21, 1924, SCOF, "Press Releases"; Wilkinson to Hunt, June 9, 1924, SCOF, "Unemployment, Wilkinson, Lupton A.," HHP, HHPL.

123. Memorandum of E. E. Hunt, "Economic Investigations," June 17, 1927, SCOF, "Hunt, E. E., 1923-1928," HHP, HHPL. Hoover, foreword to *Seasonal Operation in the Construction Industries* (Washington, 1924).

124. *Annual Report of the Secretary of Commerce*, 1925, pp. 14-15.

125. Hoover, *Memoirs*, 2:101, 103.

126. Hoover to Harding, May 4, 1922, SCOF, "Twelve-Hour Day," HHP, HHPL.

127. Harding to Hoover, May 10, 1922, SCOF, "Twelve-Hour Day," HHP,

HHPL; Hoover, *Memoirs*, 2:103. There is a long discussion of this affair in Robert Zieger's *The Republicans and Labor, 1919-29*, pp. 98-108.

128. Hoover to John V. W. Reynders, May 22, 1922, SCOF, "Twelve-Hour Day," HHP, HHPL; Hoover, *Memoirs*, 2:103-4.

129. Ibid.; Hoover, Address before the National Conference of Social Work, June 27, 1922, 245, Public Statements, HHP, HHPL.

130. Hoover to Harding, November 1, 1922, SCOF, "Twelve-Hour Day," HHP, HHPL; Hoover, *Memoirs*, 2:104.

131. Ibid.

132. Hoover to Harding, May 26, 1923, and June 13, 1923; Harding to Hoover, June 18, 1923, SCOF, "Twelve-Hour Day," HHP, HHPL.

133. Elbert H. Gary to Harding, June 27, 1923, SCOF, "Twelve-Hour Day," HHP, HHPL.

134. Press Release from Department of Commerce, July 5, 1923; Hoover's contribution to Harding's Tacoma Address, SCOF, "Twelve-Hour Day," HHP, HHPL; Hoover, *Memoirs*, 2:104.

135. Hoover, Address before the Boston Chamber of Commerce, March 24, 1920, 53, Public Statements; Herbert Hoover, "What America Faces," *Industrial Management*, April 1, 1921, 141, Public Statements, HHP, HHPL.

136. Materials at the Hoover Presidential Library indicate that Hoover's public relations activities in support of these concerns were limited to occasional addresses, press releases, and magazine articles prepared by his journalist friends. His efforts in these areas did not constitute concerted publicity "campaigns," and, in my view, study of them would reveal nothing new about his use of publicity as an administrative tool.

137. Hoover, Address before the National Conference of Street and Highway Safety, December 15, 1924, 422, Public Statements, HHP, HHPL.

138. Herbert Hoover, *The New Day: Campaign Speeches of Herbert Hoover, 1928*, pp. 152-53. Hoover's use of the term "American system" to describe his anti-statist political philosophy was evidently suggested to him by Edward Hunt. See Hunt's memorandum to Hoover, "The Cooperative Committee and Conference System," December 14, 1926, SCOF, "Hunt, E. E., 1923-1928," HHP, HHPL. In the memorandum, Hunt used the term in recommending that Hoover make his "committee and conference system" a permanent government "instrument."

7 An Unpopular Presidency

IN THE FALL OF 1927, the tremendous public relations apparatus that Herbert Hoover had assembled for administrative purposes was mobilized behind the administrator's presidential candidacy. As he had been urged to do for years, he now "unleashed" his publicity personnel and allowed them to sell him politically as they had once sold his Belgian relief, Food Administration, and Department of Commerce programs. George Akerson began his work in October by calling upon the assistance of Hoover's many journalist and editor friends to "mould public sentiment" behind the secretary. The valuable services of William Allen White, Mark Sullivan, and Arch Shaw were thus quickly secured. Veteran reporters Will Irwin and William Hard were contacted to write pro-Hoover articles and to prepare campaign biographies of the candidate. When completed, these works were syndicated in several press services, sent to all delegates to the Republican National Convention, and used by the Republican National Committee as propaganda after the nomination.[1]

Such old Hoover friends and associates as Raymond Mayer, George Barr Baker, Edgar Rickard, and Frederick Feiker also became integral members of the team helping Akerson and Republican National Committee publicity director Henry J. Allen to boost their "Chief's" candidacy. At Hoover's ARA and American Child Health Association office at 42 Broadway in New York, where all the administrator's past public statements had been cataloged since 1920, Baker and Rickard distributed thousands of copies of these utterances to influential editors and organizations. Under the direction of Feiker, the Associated Business Editors formed a special "Hoover for President" subcommittee, which sent out a series of pro-Hoover "bulletins" to business editors during the campaign.[2]

In addition to these longtime acquaintances, there were two influential newcomers to the Hoover publicity forces in 1928. A. H. Kirchhofer, editor of the Buffalo *News* and a member of the board of directors of the American Society of Newspaper Editors, wrote propaganda for Hoover out of the publicity headquarters of the Republican National Committee. More informally, Bruce Barton, the well-known New York public relations figure, lent a hand during the campaign. A former Coolidge speech-writer and author of such popular works as *The Man Nobody Knows* and *The Book Nobody Knows*, Barton proved an effective Hoover advocate. He issued a widely publicized rebuttal of Henry L. Mencken's iconoclastic satirization of Hoover as a "fat Coolidge." And through his friend Merle Thorpe, editor of the *Nation's Business*, Barton suggested the spirit and much of the wording of Hoover's often-quoted telegram to the Republican Convention: "You say that I have earned the right to the presidential nomination. No man can establish such an obligation upon any part of the American people. My country owes me no debt. It gave me, as it gives every boy and girl, a chance. . . . In no other land could a boy from a country village, without inheritance or influential friends, look forward with unbounded hope."[3]

In November, 1928, Hoover was elected president of the United States, receiving 21.4 million votes to Al Smith's 15.0 million and carrying forty states—including five southern states that no Republican had carried since Reconstruction. The size of this victory was not surprising; for all other political considerations aside, Hoover was the standard-bearer for the party of prosperity, and it had been easy for his many devoted propagandists to associate the active former secretary of commerce with the "creation" of that prosperity. But though it could not be seen at the time, the triumphal presidential campaign of 1928 was to be Hoover's last successful public relations drive. A brief four years later, he would find him-

self bitterly attacked in the press, the butt of cutting jokes cir-
culating throughout the country and in the Capital, and the subject of a spate of highly unscrupulous, but marketable, works
accusing him of financial dishonesty throughout his career. He
would become a disappointment even to some of his staunchest
friends and advocates. And his defeat in 1932 at the hands of
Franklin Delano Roosevelt, almost an exact reversal of his own
victory over Smith, was, it would seem, an accurate reflection of
his unpopularity in all sections of the country.[4]

In evaluating this overwhelming reversal of sentiment, it is necessary to look deeper than the mere fact of the Great Depression.
For granting the obvious effect of this in diminishing Hoover's
stature, there remains a paradox to be explained here. How was it
that a man whose whole public career had been attuned to public
opinion and the need for good relationships with the press now
lost so suddenly and so painfully the support of both the people
and the journalists? How was it that a public relations–conscious
administrator became a president so remarkable for his failure in
public relations? To answer these questions, it is necessary to examine Hoover's peculiar administrative style—and the personality
and philosophy that shaped it—in the context of a crisis-ridden
presidency.

I

Hoover came to the White House, he writes in his *Memoirs*,
"determined" to "carry forward the reconstruction and development measures in which [he] had participated as Secretary of
Commerce," to "initiate reforms in our social and business life,"
and to "reorient our foreign relations" toward the promotion of
"peace and international progress." "Instead of being able to devote [his] four years wholly to these purposes," he laments, he
found himself quickly "overtaken by the economic hurricane"
and forced to contend with the problem of "economic recovery
and employment."[5] What he fails to say, however, is that in dealing with the crucial issues of "recovery and employment," his basic

approach was essentially that used for "reconstruction and development" when he had been secretary of commerce. And it was this application of formerly successful methods in the face of a thoroughly changed social and economic situation that, ironically, began to alter Hoover's public image and thus to destroy the rapport that he had enjoyed over so many years with the American people.

In late October, 1929, eight months after Hoover's inauguration, the stock market crashed, causing reverberations throughout the economy. The president's response, though virtually identical to his response to the economic recession and unemployment crisis of eight years earlier, was nonetheless unprecedented in the annals of the American presidency. Refusing to accept the fatalism of his secretary of the treasury, Andrew Mellon, who urged that the "natural" downturn of the business cycle be allowed to run its course, Hoover embarked upon a program to resist the deflationary trend and to mitigate its effects;[6] and acting out of a lifetime of habit and years of intensifying conviction, he carried out this program by "stimulating others to action" from behind the scenes. Between November 19 and November 27, 1929, he called leaders from industry and labor to the White House for a series of conferences. At these they pledged themselves to maintain the prevailing wage rate, to hold firmly to current employment levels, and to increase construction activity; and at the termination of each conference, the president issued press releases announcing the agreement reached and forecasting an improvement in business conditions as a result of the meeting.[7] In addition, just as he had done in 1921, he contacted each of the state governors and requested that they combat unemployment by "speeding up" "road, street, [and] public building construction."[8]

Then to coordinate the efforts of the business leaders in carrying out their pledges, Hoover turned to his close friend and former Food Administration subordinate, Julius H. Barnes, now president of the United States Chamber of Commerce. Barnes, he suggested, should create an executive committee of businessmen responsible for seeing that their promises were fulfilled, and in deciding on this type of agency, he evidently had in mind the kind of general conference of industrial leaders that he had urged upon President

Harding in August, 1921, and which had seemed so successful in "stimulating the community to action" at that time. From Hoover's viewpoint, Barnes was almost a perfect choice, both because he had been a member of the earlier conference and because, as an active participant in the Hoover "boom" of 1920 and a devoted adherent of his "Chief's" "American system," he spoke, almost verbatim, the Hoover idiom of "decentralization" and "local" and "individual initiative." He also shared fully Hoover's conviction that trade associations, with which he had worked closely through the Chamber of Commerce, were essential to the maintenance of a stable, yet unregulated, economy.[9]

In early December, 1929, Barnes assembled in Washington his National Business Survey Conference, consisting of "more than 400 'key men,' representing every branch of industry, finance, trade and commerce," and designed to plan the "means of carrying out" the president's "efforts to stimulate and stabilize business."[10] Throughout his career, beginning with his creation of the "British Committee" in his 1913 fight for the Panama-Pacific Exposition, Hoover had used similar "celebrity" conferences and committees. Through them, with the coordination of national newspaper and magazine publicity, he had sought to carry his ideas to the larger constituencies represented by their members, and he planned now to use the NBSC in the same manner. Addressing its opening session, he told the businessmen that they had been invited "to create a temporary organization for the purpose of systematically spreading into industry as a whole the measures which have been taken by some of our leading industries to counteract the effect of the recent panic in the stock market." What the country needed, he argued, was reassurance that the "vast organism of production and distribution" was "fundamentally stable." He also recalled his successful efforts of the early 1920s in expanding and contracting construction work to regulate the activity of the business cycle. These, he felt, had demonstrated the effectiveness of "the greatest tool which our economic system affords for the establishment of stability," and accordingly, he urged business leaders to expand both in the country at large and "in all branches of industry."[11] Subsequently, in the course of the next year and a half, he would repeat this call for expanded construction many times, and both he and Barnes would supplement these efforts with many optimistic public assessments of the improvement in business that was allegedly taking place.[12]

As the NBSC pursued its difficult tasks of maintaining wages and stimulating construction in the private sector of the economy, Hoover, in October, 1930, created another voluntary committee, this time to organize relief for the jobless.[13] In purpose and key personnel, the new agency was virtually identical to the Woods committee that Hoover had called into being at the close of the Conference on Unemployment in 1921. Again, Hoover's old friend, Colonel Arthur Woods, was chairman. Again, his longtime aide, Edward Hunt, was secretary; and again, as in the case of the 1921 unemployment crusade, the president arranged for the committee to operate out of the Department of Commerce, now administered by Robert P. Lamont, and to use the department's publicity facilities, still directed by Paul Croghan.[14] Instead of Lupton A. Wilkinson, however, Hoover now retained Edward Bernays to handle public relations; and it was Bernays who gave the agency its official title, the President's Emergency Committee for Employment.[15]

In methods, too, PECE operated along the same lines that the Woods committee had a decade earlier. Following the president's dictates, it functioned as a "clearing house of ideas on unemployment and relief"[16] and, to transmit these ideas, used agencies similar to those employed in 1921. To begin with, for example, there was a thirty-member central committee in Washington consisting of figures from industry, business, and the professions, which sought, in Woods's words, to bring to the "individual governor, or mayor, or chairman of a committee . . . any information . . . result[ing from] the experience of other cities so as to help the local committees, mayors or chairmen in their work."[17] In short, it served in the same function that Woods's less prestigious "field men" had served in during the fall and winter of 1921-22. Second, there were some 3,000 local PECE committees, which in theory were supposed to carry out the suggestions that the central organization offered in the reams of letters, pamphlets, and magazine articles that it sent them. Third, there was a vast public relations campaign to enlist public support, one that had Bernays and Croghan feeding materials to advertising, motion picture, and radio companies; Frederick Feiker, a member of PECE's Advisory Committee in Public Relations, lending the services of the Associated Business Papers; and Hoover's always cooperative writer friends William Hard and Marie Brown Meloney contributing their time and energy. Finally, there was a "Woman's Division," headed by Lillian D. Gillbreth and Alice M. Dickson, the former a Hoover associate in Belgian relief, the latter in his housing and child health concerns. Their agency organized "Spruce Up Your Home" and "Spruce Up Your Garden" campaigns,[18] activities that were quite similar to the "clean up" campaign of 1921.

In spite of all their activity, however, both NBSC and PECE died quietly and unproductively in the late spring of 1931. By that time, the president was at odds with Woods and especially with Bernays, who had become highly critical of the almost total reliance on words without action.[19] As early as December, 1930, both he and Woods had begun pressing for stronger executive action, increased public works, and "a real set of objectives." Without these things, he felt, PECE had been left "up in the air," with its members and the president under the "unlimited self-delusion" that they were accomplishing something through exhortation.[20]

Why did Hoover not respond to such criticism from within and move in the direction of enlarged federal authority and new governmental responsibilities? A part of the explanation appears to lie in the fact that after almost thirty years of orchestrating national publicity and committee activity, this type of administrative approach had become virtually ingrained. In the beginning, to be sure, during his campaigns for the Panama-Pacific Exposition and the CRB, he had regarded it as being purely instrumental. But during the Food Administration years, he had come to view it as more than a matter of practicality or expediency. It became for him the servant of a strongly held political point of view, the way, in other words, to implement the ideal of decentralized authority with its moral virtues of individual initiative and responsibility; and after seven years of successful coordination of public relations and committee work as secretary of commerce, he was ap-

parently convinced that this was the only type of administration
consistent with the "American system." Wedded to it now by temperament and political conviction, convinced, moreover, that it
had been eminently "constructive" for a quarter of a century, he
could do no other than apply it and persist in it as president.

Hoover's faith in his "theory of administration," i.e., centralized
decision-making and decentralized execution, had been frequently affirmed in his campaign speeches.[21] During his presidency,
this faith remained unshakable, the chief executive asserting it
time and again in his public statements. In October, 1930, a week
before announcing the creation of PECE, he stated, for example,
that the country's social and economic well-being had been, and
would continue to be, dependent upon the "American system."
For him, "tendencies of communities and states to shirk their own
responsibilities or to unload them on the Federal government"
were "destructive" of the American "pattern of self-government."
In his view, it was "the first duty of those who believe in the American system to maintain a knowledge and pride in it. . . ."[22] Ten
months later, the president organized a new unemployment relief
organization to carry on the work of the now defunct PECE. In
spite of the internal criticisms of Bernays and Woods, the president could say at this time: "I cannot speak too highly of the actual
results obtained by the multitude of committees and the public
authorities over last winter."[23] As late as July, 1932, in urging the
continuation of PECE's successor, the Organization on Unemployment Relief, he remained convinced of the rightness of his old
methods:

> This organization is comprised of leading men and women
> throughout every state in the Union. . . . [It] is the only
> agency for national coordination and stimulation for the multi-
> tude of voluntary efforts. . . . Voluntary effort amongst our
> people is of far more importance both morally and financially
> than the direct aid of local or other governmental agencies.[24]

In his addresses of this period, Hoover was fond of saying that if
the nation clung to its institutions and ideals during the economic
crisis, those institutions and ideals would emerge stronger than
ever after the emergency had passed. He had expressed the same

sentiment as food administrator during World War I and as secretary of commerce during the unemployment crisis of 1921.

In the economic chaos following the stock market crash, however, the Hoover public relations strategy of "educating the community to its responsibilities," of "stimulating it to action," of "building public confidence," and of relying upon voluntary cooperation could not work. When used before, improvements had seemed to follow, at least as a matter of coincidence if not result. But now they did not, and in a period marked by the growing insolvency of local institutions, palpably falling construction levels and wage rates, and rising unemployment,[25] the administration's continued insistence on local voluntarism and its optimistic evaluations of the situation opened up a wide credibility gap between observable reality and official assessment. Within two years of his inauguration, Hoover's persistent efforts to combat the depression by "assisting others to action" rather than committing the resources of the federal government had begun to cut heavily into the storehouse of public good will that he had accumulated over the years.

A decline in stature, to be sure, would have attended any man confronted with the economic disaster of the early 1930s. But Hoover's fall was especially precipitous, for the public had expected him to meet and overcome the challenge as he had seemed to do so often in the past. Ironically, although his public relations style was actually a manifestation of a "retiring" personality and a "weak" political philosophy, the image that his publicists had created was quite the opposite. They had not, as he had urged, "kept his name out of" administrative publicity. On the contrary, impressed with Hoover as the hardest-working and most devoted public official of the Harding and Coolidge administrations and charmed by his modesty, they had written of him as "America's handyman," a commanding figure who "acted while others talked," and one whose expertise enabled him to act with "facts" in hand on a dozen economic and social problems.[26] During the campaign of 1928, they had been careful to remind the public of his wartime relief work and his handling of the Mississippi flood. Will Irwin, for example, had produced a motion picture, "The Master of Emergencies," from old CRB, ARA, and Mississippi flood film footage. A number of copies of the movie had been distributed across the country for showings by Republican organizations. Through efforts such as these, the image of a "master of emergencies" was deliberately laid upon that of the resourceful "social engineer."[27] Charles Evans Hughes, who had delivered many pro-Hoover campaign speeches, including an election eve appeal over nationwide radio, had once stated what many Americans were quite ready to believe: "If any difficult situation should arise, the man who more than any one else could be depended upon to bring the widest knowledge and the greatest resourcefulness to the devising of means to meet the emergency would be Herbert Hoover."[28]

Thus, when Hoover came to the presidency, it was the "practical" component of his 1920 image of "practical idealist" that had been underscored by his publicists.[29] Not projected nearly so much were his more deeply rooted "idealist" tendency and the almost religious intensity with which he valued "individualism" and its political corollaries, "local initiative and responsibility." Some of the phrasing of Hoover's statements of the 1920s had seemed to suggest a strong pragmatic bent to his mind and social outlook. He had said on occasion that *"words without action are the assassins of idealism"* (Hoover's emphasis) or, again, that "wisdom does not so much consist of knowledge of the ultimate, it consists of knowing what to do next."[30] However, these expressions of the "engineering-scientific" side of his personality had always been undercut by his dogmatic faith in "American Individualism" and by the "American system," which constituted for him, in fact, a kind of ultimate truth. Proud of his Quaker church for holding "the most strongly individualistic concept of any of the churches," Hoover had referred to the sentiments expressed in *American Individualism* as his "gospel." His public addresses on "American Individualism" he had referred to as "preaching sermons," and he had urged copies of *American Individualism* on his friends as being "good for their souls."[31] How this absolutist, religious bent of mind had wrestled with, and finally cancelled out, the "pragmatic" tendency is made clear in two short illogical sentences from *American Individualism*: "We cannot ever afford to rest at ease in the comfortable assumption that right ideas always prevail by some virtue of their own. In the long run they do."[32]

After his nomination, Hoover himself had begun to worry about his distorted public image. To Ray T. Tucker, a reporter in his campaign entourage, he had remarked that he hoped his campaign speeches would help "live down his reputation as an engineer."[33] Then, after his election, his fears had grown. Apprehensive, as he had always been before undertaking a new administrative challenge, he had complained to his old friend Willis J. Abbot that he had been "over-advertised": "My friends have made the American people think of me as a sort of a superman, able to cope successfully with the most difficult and complicated problems. They expect the impossible of me and should there arise in the land conditions with which the political machinery is unable to cope, I will be the one to suffer."[34] With his entry into the White House, he would find his lifelong apprehensions, finally and devastatingly, justified. Answering the economic crisis as only personality, conscience, and past administrative experience would allow, it was not long before the discrepancy between the "ideal" Hoover and the "real" one became conspicuous.

It was this discrepancy, of course, that the Democratic party propagandist Charles Michelson was soon exploiting, quite consciously and with deadly effect.[35] It also became a favorite theme of other journalists. Walter Lippmann wrote in June, 1930, "By arousing certain expectations, the [Hoover] legend has established a standard by which the public has estimated him; if, as I think most observers would admit, his first year ended in an atmosphere of mild disappointment, the cause in some measure was the inability of the real Hoover to act up to the standards of the ideal Hoover."[36] A year and a half later Elliott Thurston made a similar comment. "Mr. Hoover," he said, "permitted himself to be advertised as the master mind, the superman, the engineering genius who had grappled successfully with the biggest, hardest problems in modern times. . . . Badly oversold . . . the contrast between the advertising . . . and what he has been able to deliver [has been] conspicuous to the point of painfulness."[37]

II

Victimized by a false public image that his habitual privateness and concealment had inadvertently helped to prepare, Hoover's

rapid fall from public esteem was also facilitated by the notori-
ously bad relationship that developed between his administration
and the Washington press corps. A year after taking office, these
relations had become so bad that Fred Fuller Shedd, president of
the American Society of Newspaper Editors (a group whose board
of directors included Hoover's close friends William Allen White,
David Lawrence, Willis Abbot, and A. H. Kirchhofer), felt that
the president's only hope in "getting his story before the public"
was to reach "beyond the Washington correspondents" to the editors.[38] Seventeen months later, the situation had gone from bad to
worse. In October, 1931, Washington correspondent Paul Anderson, a Hoover admirer during the 1920s, asserted:

> The relations of Herbert Hoover with the newspapermen whose
> work brings them in immediate contact with the Presidential
> office have reached a stage of unpleasantness without parallel
> during the present century. They are characterized by mutual
> dislike, unconcealed suspicion, and downright bitterness. This
> ugly condition has frequently been reflected in the utterances
> of the President and the conduct of his aides, and is bound to be
> reflected in some of the news dispatches, although to nothing like
> the extent of its actual existence.[39]

If only partially "reflected in [their] news dispatches," the bitterness of some correspondents toward the president was fully revealed in their magazine articles and books. They referred to him
sarcastically as the "Big," "Great," or "Super Administrator," "The
Strong Silent Leader," or the "Big Executive."[40] For correspondent
Ray Tucker, once a warm supporter of Hoover's candidacy and
admirer of his press relations,[41] the White House had become a
"grim and efficient center where the Great Engineer labors. . . ."
Writing anonymously, he now saw fit to depict the president as
"fretful and feeble," a "victim of self-pity" ("our first hairshirt
hero"), as "dynamic as a 30 watt bulb," and a leader who sur-
rounded himself with "sychophantic counsellors" and interposed
between himself and the press "couriers, courtiers, and second-
hand interviewers." These qualities, Tucker felt, explained the
massive "defection of the young and idealistic members of the
Washington corp of correspondents."[42]

In the eyes of other journalists, Hoover was condemned as a "Super-Babbitt," who had not simply been oversold by others (as Hoover himself was aware), but who had been doing the "selling" himself for decades.[43] "Not for a minute would I deny his [Hoover's] great skill as a ballyhoo artist," wrote Heywood Broun. "Upon retirement from the White House there is no reason why he should not obtain a lucrative position in one of our great advertising agencies. He performed an extraordinary feat first of all in selling himself."[44] Robert Allen, now collaborating in secrecy with Drew Pearson, agreed with Broun. The president, he charged, was "one of the super-promoters of the age," a man who had been able "by a consummate sense of publicity to create the illusion of heroism and greatness and to attain world acclaim," but one who lacked "the essential requisites of character to enact the role he had created."[45] Some of this criticism, of course, particularly that directed at Hoover's unshakable public relations strategy of "confidence-building" public statements, conferences, and commissions, was readily understandable. Given the desperate social situation, such an approach seemed more and more inadequate. But how was it that a man who had successfully cultivated the friendship of the press for three decades, now that he needed this friendship more than ever, should inspire such acerbic and unfair *ad hominem* attacks? To answer this question, it is necessary to look closely at another but often neglected side of Hoover's press relations.

Hoover had begun his presidency, as he had all his previous administrations, by expressing in his first presidential press conference, held the day after his inauguration, his desire for cordial relations with the correspondents. After pledging to meet with them personally twice a week and to make available his press secretary, George Akerson, on a daily basis, he had further pleased them by promising to liberalize the press conference procedure and permit more direct quotation than had been allowed by previous presidents.[46] This would be done, he had said, within the framework of a tripartite system, one that had been suggested to him by his friend and veteran White House correspondent Mark Sullivan, whose advice he had solicited on the matter. In addition to the more frequent statements that could be directly quoted, other statements would be given out only for attribution to "the White House," or only for "background." Sullivan, as his memorandum on the subject makes clear, had regarded this as simply a continuation of the normal procedure used by past presidents;[47] but the manner in which Hoover had presented it gave the universal impression that he had completely abolished the "trial balloon" device of the "White House spokesman."[48] Consequently, when he failed to do this, correspondents were surprised and resentful. They would not have been, perhaps, had they been more perceptive of the Hoover personality in the years before he came to the White House.

Awed by Hoover's administrative gifts and appreciative of his accessibility and his great value to them as a "grapevine," reporters in the 1920s had tended to discount certain negative character traits that became magnified during his presidency. In particular, they had been willing to ignore or tolerate his self-righteous sense of the superiority of his own judgment and, related to this, his great sensitivity to criticism. At times during this earlier period, even though his attentiveness to public opinion had made him cognizant of the need for friends in the press, he had reacted with extreme bitterness when a writer, editor, or newspaper had criticized or, as Hoover put it, "misrepresented" his position. Such "misrepresentation," he had fretted on several occasions, unless acknowledged publicly by its perpetrators, would prevent "decent men from going into public service."[49] In reality, it seems, because of his strong self-image as the man above politics working unselfishly for the commonweal from behind the scenes, he tended to see the journalists not as "partners," as he sometimes said, but as subordinates who should do his bidding to help him to serve the public. He could not and never did appreciate their role as social critics as well as reporters. And most of the correspondents, apparently admiring Hoover too much to realize this, had tolerated both his "thin-skin" and the various measures he had taken as secretary of commerce to regulate all news items passing out of his news-conscious department.[50] This tolerance began to dissipate quickly after he became president.

Portents of the open antagonism that would develop between

Hoover and the press had actually begun to surface during the 1928 campaign and during Hoover's postelection good-will trip to Latin America. Listening to Hoover expatiate on current affairs in his Department of Commerce office or press room, the reporters had not been fully aware of his painful shyness and the degree to which he protected his personal privacy, traits that would soon compound the difficulties inherent in his inability to bear criticism or "unauthorized" reporting. During the campaign, however, these traits had become more obvious, especially when correspondents found it almost impossible to cover or to photograph the candidate or to find materials for "human interest" stories about him. This was true even in Hoover's hometown, West Branch, Iowa, where the bewildered reporters, expecting a field day for "hokum," could scarcely locate the candidate.[51] On the Latin American tour, moreover, press doubts about continued good relations with Hoover had been further heightened by his designation of his long-time press aide, George Barr Baker, to handle the radio dispatches of the eighteen correspondents who were traveling with him on the *U.S.S. Maryland.* That Baker had been a naval censor during World War I and had used his training to abridge the contents of their releases seemed an ominous sign to many journalists.[52]

Though these doubts abated briefly after the president's promises to liberalize press conference procedures, they soon reappeared and before long had been transformed into an abiding hostility. Symptomatic of what was to come were two articles that appeared in the newspaper trade journal *Editor and Publisher* in July, 1929, both bearing complaints against Hoover that would soon become quite familiar. Written by George Manning, the Washington correspondent for the journal, they charged, first of all, that instead of the hoped for "liberalization" of press methods, there had been "a general 'tightening up.' " Hoover, in other words, had been angered by the contents of true but unfavorable stories. He had decided to punish the authors; and, as a result, his administration was charging certain correspondents with writing false or unauthorized stories and was applying pressure, through their news service chiefs or editors, to have them fired. Drew Pearson had also "found himself faced with being barred from every office of the government," although the threat had not actually been carried out. Whether Hoover was really behaving in this way is a question that cannot be answered from the surviving documents in his presidential papers, but given the fact that he had acted similarly as secretary of commerce,[53] it seems quite likely that he was. In any case, the newspapermen believed that he had used, and was continuing to use, such tactics against their colleagues, and the result was suspicion and resentment that never abated.[54]

There were also two other major complaints voiced in Manning's articles. One alleged that Hoover's press conferences, instead of producing "real" news and quotable copy, had degenerated into a system by which the president disseminated propagandistic "handouts," thus making the newsmen mere purveyors of the administration's "line."[55] The other claimed that Hoover was deliberately thwarting the legitimate function of the press to cover the president, not only by barring them from his weekend mountain retreat in Virginia, but also by preventing them from following his progress to and from the "Rapidan Camp."[56]

Such complaints became increasingly bitter after the stock market crash and the onset of the depression.[57] Hoover, it seemed, was now more determined than ever to maintain secrecy and privacy; and consequently, except for a few privileged correspondents—William Hard and Mark Sullivan, who were members of the "medicine ball cabinet,"—members of the Washington press corps could obtain little reliable information on presidential activities, official or unofficial. Forced to speculate or to rely on unauthorized sources in composing their stories, they repeatedly incurred the wrath of the president and his secretaries, George Akerson, Theodore Joslin, and Lawrence Richey, for filing erroneous or "frivolous" reports.[58] And antagonized by this, they responded in kind, taking out their resentment on the president, his aides, and the few "fair-haired" boys who enjoyed the special privileges denied to the rest of them.[59] Presidential press relations, it appeared, were caught in a vicious downward spiral; and as the spiral descended, the new depression image of Hoover as hardhearted reactionary began to be fixed in the public mind.

As Hoover's press relations deteriorated, friends and well-wishers of the president sent warnings and advice. One comment, for example, came from Karl A. Bickel, president of the United Press Association and a Hoover supporter, who, in sending a copy of the first Manning article to George Akerson by way of a mutual friend, noted that "an unhealthy situation rather full of potentialities" was being created. "Nobody is ever going to control, mould, direct or shape the press in this country," he declared. "That road has been tentatively explored before with inevitably bad results."[60] Akerson, though agreeing that it was a matter "that should be gone into," brushed off Manning's charges as "just an alibi for five or six things that have happened where the newspaper profession has been at fault itself."[61] A year later, A. H. Kirchhofer, an important Hoover publicity director during the 1928 campaign, sent the president a fifteen-page single-spaced memorandum, noting that he was "grieved, as I am sure you must be, that [Washington correspondents] who in the past were friendly . . . have become critics," and that something should be done to "re-establish the friendly relations which prevailed at the Commerce Department." Hoover, he continued, could make friends if he would "just give the rank and file something to write about." And by this, he explained:

> I don't mean quotes. Give them the idea about what you are doing and enough background information so they can interpret the administration on some of those things. That would keep your aims and accomplishments before the public—all the time. If you haven't the time to think about this, surely there is some one in the White House who can. I think it is as important as anything you can do. . . . You've had popular support before in unlimited quantity. I think you need it now and surely you need it for the future. Pardon me for saying I do not believe the methods used since your election will accomplish it.[62]

The president, in other words, should spend more time with representatives of the press, be more open with them, and let both them and the country know that he was not an "automaton."[63]

Though Hoover briefly replied to Kirchhofer, thanking him for his "helpful" remarks, the advice proferred by the latter could only fall on deaf ears.[64] Hard-pressed in meeting ever new developments in the economic crisis, he felt that he could not afford to spend more time with members of the press corps,[65] nor was he inclined to be more "open" with them. This, he seemed to think, might engender the spread of confidence-destroying "leaks" or rumors, thus delaying what was to him the key to economic recovery, the restoration of "psychological confidence."[66] As we have seen, he had long believed that "psychology" was a key factor in determining levels of economic activity;[67] and now, just as he had done as secretary of commerce, he tried to build confidence through the use of optimistic press releases.[68] This time, however, the strategy was not working, and for this, he tended to blame an uncooperative press rather than any defect in his approach. To prevent "sabotage" of his efforts, he retreated into secrecy, conducted his presidential business in unannounced conferences and over the telephone in the privacy of his office,[69] and became increasingly guarded in dealing with journalists. Holding fewer and fewer press conferences as his term ran its course, he was no longer a "grapevine" for them. Yet all the while, he kept insisting that they should become more cooperative, that, in particular, they should "express the justified optimism of American business, industry, and agriculture."[70] To longtime friends in the press corps, he requested the cancellation of stories and even the suppression of news, all in the name of "psychological confidence."[71]

For a man of Hoover's temperament and ideology, then, the counsel that Kirchhofer had given could not truly be "helpful." The president could not change "his ways," and the press would not accept the role that he had assigned to it. It would not become simply a purveyor of official optimism. What had once been a two-way relationship between Hoover and the journalists had now become a one-way relationship, and the rift that had opened in July, 1929, merely widened thereafter.[72]

III

With the "channel to the public mind" provided by the press thus obstructed, Hoover's aides and friends—men such as Arthur Woods, William Hard, William Allen White, Willis Abbot, and

David Lawrence—urged him to use the radio to take his case to the public.[73] In sharp contrast, however, with a man like Richard M. Nixon, who was to build his political career by "shortcircuiting" a hostile press,[74] Hoover was simply incapable of "going over it" by making direct appeals to the nation. Temperamentally unsuited to public exposure, he had, throughout his career, functioned behind the scenes, "reaching out to the public" through the mobilization of the printed media and committee organization. And though he had felt compelled to give many addresses during the 1920s, he had never enjoyed doing so, and the speeches had been delivered mechanically with his face deflected downward into his text.[75] During his presidency, his speaking ability did not improve, and apparently he was convinced that not much could be done to improve it.[76] He had warned his supporters that they could never make "a Teddy Roosevelt" out of him. Now, when urged to dramatize his leadership, he would invariably reply, "This is not a showman's job. I will not step out of character."[77]

With the president temperamentally unable to refurbish his public image, yet desirous of succeeding himself in the White House,[78] the virtually impossible task of "reselling" him to the American public fell heavily on the shoulders of his advisers and friends. Receiving little help from Hoover, who, though stung by the criticisms hurled at him, characteristically preferred to remain passive rather than launch a public counterattack,[79] his press secretaries, George Akerson and Theodore Joslin, attempted to "humanize" the president by bringing to public attention the qualities that they had long found so endearing and that had inspired their loyalty. In a national radio broadcast in June, 1930, Akerson informed the public about "how the President of the United States fills his day"; and later, in replying to a friend who had urged more such "human interest" material, he lamented that there was a "natural hesitancy on the part of those who are working directly under [the President] to act as a spokesman." "Some one of these days," he said, "I want to have a talk with you about this whole problem of humanizing."[80] Joslin, who replaced Akerson in March, 1931, after the latter had taken a public relations job with Paramount Films, encountered similar difficulties. Again, he had to fight the president's deeply rooted abhorrence to "personal publicity"; and, as a result, his efforts to "humanize" him were so obvious that they produced as much ridicule as praise.[81] Supplementing the abortive efforts of Akerson and Joslin, Hoover's lifelong friends and celebrators Will Irwin and Vernon Kellogg also tried to interpret his "mysterious" personality to a now skeptical American public. And finally, French Strother, now serving as the president's speechwriting assistant, drafted a paper on "The Personality of President Hoover" published under the name of the recent secretary of commerce, Robert Lamont.[82] Given the president's continued public silence and inaccessibility, however, none of these efforts did much to revive his popularity.

Hoover's seclusion and the consequent lack of coordination between him and his aides is perhaps the best explanation, too, for the two incredible public relations gaffes of his administration. One of these had Akerson first telling the press that Justice Harlan F. Stone was the Hoover nominee for chief justice of the Supreme Court, then reading a formal statement from the president announcing the nomination of Charles Evans Hughes. The other was the issuance by the White House of the "Conclusions and Recommendations" of the Wickersham Commission report, a version that was almost diametrically opposed to the views of a majority of the commissioners.[83] The "distance" between Hoover and his staff may also explain their inept and ineffective publicity of an overtly political nature. In the fall of 1930, for instance, David Hinshaw, a presidential assistant, founded in cooperation with the Republican National Committee a newspaper entitled *Washington: A Journal of Information and Opinion Concerning the Operation of Our National Government.* Its purpose, so its promoters said, was to impress Hoover's achievements upon Republican precinct workers and thus enable them to offset criticism of the president during the off-year elections.[84] Yet, if this was the purpose, the first issue proved to be a peculiar piece of exhortation, dwelling, as it did, on the "handicaps of Hoover," the foremost of which was frankly identified as his "inability to talk in the political vernacular" and thus to "lead the American people."[85] Moreover, as the Democrats gleefully discovered, the issue that bore this dubious charge to the troops had been printed in a Maryland shop owned by one of the state's Democratic politicians. The second issue, needless to say, did contain Hoover-championing articles by Will Irwin and William Allen White and was struck off in another printery. But this establishment, it was discovered, was an "open shop" unaffiliated with the Typographical Union of America; and fearful of political repercussions, the president finally ordered that the five and one-half tons of freshly printed copy should be destroyed. The third issue of the ill-fated venture, published on November 15, 1930, opened with an editorial announcing the demise of the paper because of a lack of subscriptions. "Perhaps," it was admitted, "our execution of the idea—continuously to widen the circle of informed public opinion—has not been good enough; perhaps the time is out of joint; perhaps, after all, the idea [has not been] too good."[86]

Such amateurish and uncoordinated political publicity was characteristic of Hoover's presidency. There was difference of opinion and bickering between his own longtime publicists and the Republican National Committee over how to deal with Charles Michelson, the troublesome Democratic publicist. In September, 1930, a committee member urged George Barr Baker to exert his influence to end "the humiliating and ridiculous situation" that found Republican propagandists preoccupied with proving Michelson "a liar," rather than ignoring him and playing up the president's "constructive proposals."[87] Later, Baker himself and Edgar Rickard were scolding Republican National Chairman Robert H. Lucas for unjustly accusing Michelson of promoting James O'Brien's smear biography, *Hoover's Millions and How He Made Them.* Feeling that Democrats perhaps more than Republicans had repudiated the book, Baker charged Lucas with committing "a serious error" in failing to give credit "to our opponents when they play a sporting game with us."[88] But the problem was greater than disunity among Hoover's publicists. As Kirchhofer had pointed out to the president, his propagandists were simply too unimaginative to be effective. One "excellent example" of amateurish approach, he said, was announcing that "a campaign to sell the administration's achievements was to be undertaken." "The expert," Kirchhofer noted, "would go ahead and tell his

stories, as if no pre-conceived plan were involved. The announcement is a warning to watch out for the ballyhoo." The anti-ad-
ministration propaganda, he continued, as disseminated by Michelson, was much more effective; and the administration, he
thought, should adopt similar tactics.[89]

Such counsel, however, went unheeded. Fifteen months later,
Kirchhofer was once again urging upon the president "a radical
revision of certain White House publicity methods, or perhaps it
would be better to say attitudes. . . ." Implicitly critical now of
the president himself, he argued that James West, the man recently chosen by Hoover to counteract Democratic publicity, "hadn't
a chance against Michelson," partly because, unlike those of the
latter, "every effort he makes has to be submitted to editing"[90] and
partly because he was primarily a "reporter," not a publicity agent.
A more effective man, Kirchhofer implied, would be Raymond
Mayer, the former Lupton A. Wilkinson vice-president and Hoover publicist in 1928. Such a man, he felt, would know "the difference between straight news reporting and writing publicity or
propaganda"; and there was, in his opinion, "a vast difference."[91]
Despite Kirchhofer's considered advice, both West and Akerson,
the latter returning to his "Chief's" side for the 1932 campaign,
were key figures in Hoover's unsuccessful bid for reelection.[92] And
once again, their work, mirroring the Hoover campaign as a whole,
was uninspired and undistinguished. As an analyst of the 1932
campaign has written:

> The most consistently used strategem employed by the [Republi-
> can] publicity bureau to enhance Mr. Hoover's prospects in 1932
> was represented by those 'prosperity just around the corner'
> predictions and 'the worst has passed' statements. These . . .
> utterances, so multiform in number and so uniform in character,
> were proved exceedingly silly as time passed. They did more
> harm than good. They played squarely into the Democratic
> hands and . . . made Mr. Hoover a scapegoat upon whom
> everybody blamed everything.[93]

IV

In assessing Hoover's calamitous fall from public esteem, then,
one must conclude that, once the stock market crash had occurred,

he was as much a victim of his own behind-the-scenes, public relations style of administration as he was of the ensuing depression. Having fashioned a publicity-oriented mode of administrative procedure to fit the unique requirements of his personality and philosophy, he had risen to the presidency, almost without design, on the strength of a "grass roots" popularity indirectly produced by his techniques. Yet, once in the office, he was confronted with problems that called for a quite different approach, one that his temperament, philosophical convictions, and lack of political skills made virtually impossible for him to adopt. Reacting as only personality, philosophy, and past experience would permit, he applied the same techniques and approach that he had used successfully in the past. But this time they failed. In the lonely isolation of the White House, Hoover's lifelong fears of failure became reality; and ironically, the sense of this was heightened by the image of "master of emergencies" and "social engineer" that his public relations style had created for him. Under the warping pressures of a crisis-dominated presidency, moreover, the traits that had moulded this style and so terribly unsuited him for the times—his distaste, in other words, for public exposure, his inability to dramatize his leadership, his dogmatic individualism and antistatism, his sensitivity to criticism—were painfully revealed for all, even his closest friends,[94] to see; and under the new set of circumstances, such characteristics only antagonized the press, confused and frustrated his aides, publicists, and advisers, and made him all the more unpopular. An effective publicizer of causes throughout his career, Hoover thus saw his own presidency become, paradoxically, a public relations disaster and the White House, truly, "a compound hell."[95]

1.   George Akerson to William Allen White, October 10, 1927, George E. Akerson Papers, HHPL; "William Hard," "Mark Sullivan," and "Arch Shaw," White House Secretary Files—George Akerson, Presidential Papers, HHP, HHPL; Will Irwin to Christian Herter, November 16, 1927; Irwin to Akerson, December 21, 1927, Akerson Papers, HHPL; Memorandum, A. H. Kirchhofer to Hoover, "Publicity," August 24, 1928, Campaign and Pre-Inaugural Papers, 1928-1929, HHP, HHPL.

2.   "Ray Mayer," White House Secretary Files—George Akerson, Presidential Papers, HHP, HHPL; Baker to Akerson, April 18, 1928; Akerson to Edgar Rick-

ard, April 7, 1928, and May 2, 1928, Akerson Papers, HHPL; "National Republican Committee Department Heads," (Memorandum), n.d., Campaign and Pre-Inaugural Papers, 1928-1929, HHP, HHPL; Feiker to Hoover, July 2, 1928; "Nine Years at Hoover's Elbow," Feiker Papers, General Accessions, HHPL; "Hoover for President," Business Paper Editorial Advisory Committee, Campaign and Pre-Inaugural Papers, 1928-1929, HHP, HHPL.

3.   Herbert Hoover, *The New Day*, p. 3; Bruce Barton to Hoover (with enclosure), September 7, 1928, Campaign and Pre-Inaugural Papers, 1928-1929, HHP, HHPL; Barton to Merle Thorpe (with enclosures), May 19, 1928, Box 28, Hoover File, Bruce Barton Papers, University of Wisconsin.

4.   Hoover polled 15.8 million votes to Roosevelt's 22.8 million. He was able to carry but six states.

5.   Herbert Hoover, *The Memoirs of Herbert Hoover: The Cabinet and the Presidency, 1920-1933*, 2:223.

6.   Herbert Hoover, *The Memoirs of Herbert Hoover: The Great Depression, 1929-1941*, 3:30-32.

7.   See press statements numbered 75, 76, and 77 in Herbert Hoover, *The State Papers and Other Public Writings of Herbert Hoover*, ed. William S. Myers, 1:133-36; Hoover, *Memoirs*, 2:42-43; Albert U. Romasco, *The Poverty of Abundance: Hoover, the Nation, the Depression*, (New York, 1965), pp. 27-29. Romasco's book, though published too early to be informed by the papers at the Hoover Presidential Library, remains the best work on Hoover as president. I have found it a very instructive and helpful guide in carrying out my own inquiry.

8.   Telegram to Governors of the States, Statement 78, in Hoover, *State Papers*, 1:137.

9.   Hoover to Julius Barnes, November 15, 1929, Presidential Papers, Presidential Personal File, HHP, HHPL; Press Statement 76, in Hoover, *State Papers*, 1:136; Romasco, *The Poverty of Abundance*, pp. 29-30; Edward Eyre Hunt, *Report of the President's Conference on Unemployment* (Washington, 1921), p. 7.

10.   Press release published in New York *Times*, December 6, 1929, and cited in Romasco, *The Poverty of Abundance*, p. 30.

11.   Address, Statement 82, in Hoover, *State Papers*, 1:181-84.

12.   In addition to the exhortations of Hoover and Barnes for expanded construction, a National Survey Building Conference was created in late January, 1930, for the special purpose of convincing the public via the mass media, that conditions were "especially favorable" for new building. This committee, formed under the auspices of the National Business Survey Conference, was immediately recognized by *Business Week* for what it was: a committee "to make propaganda" (Romasco, *The Poverty of Abundance*, pp. 45-55).

13.   Press Statement 169, in Hoover, *State Papers*, I, 401.

14.   "Diary of Colonel Arthur Woods," October 23, 24, 1930, and February 26, 1931, General Accessions, HHP, HHPL; Edward Bernays, *Biography of An Idea: Memoirs of Public Relations Counsel Edward L. Bernays*, pp. 465-67; Hoover, *Memoirs*, 3:53-54.

15.   Bernays, *Biography of an Idea*, pp. 465-66.

16.   [Publicity Statement of Arthur Woods on Behalf of PECE], October, 1930, General Accessions, HHP, HHPL.

17.   Quoted in Romasco, *The Poverty of Abundance*, p. 146.

18.   "Minutes of the First Meeting of the Advisory Committee on Public Rela-

tions," 1-8, December 2, 1930; Woods's Memorandum, "Specifications and Copy Requirements for Advertising Campaign for PECE," 1-4, December 13, 1930, General Accessions; "Commerce Department Press Releases," January 8, 1931, March 16, 1931, March 18, 1931, March 21, 1931, and March 29, 1931; Alice M. Dickson to Lawrence Richey (with enclosures), April 7, 1931, Presidential Papers Official File; "Diary of Colonel Arthur Woods," General Accessions, HHP, HHPL; Romasco, *The Poverty of Abundance*, pp. 143-49.

19. Bernays, *The Biography of an Idea*, pp. 463, 466, 470-71.

20. Ibid., pp. 470-71.

21. Hoover, *The New Day*, pp. 44, 59, 78, 108, 152.

22. Hoover, *State Papers*, 1:400.

23. Ibid., 1:609-11.

24. Ibid., 2:220-21.

25. Romasco, *The Poverty of Abundance*, pp. 51-65, 148-72.

26. See, for instance, representative pro-Hoover pieces by journalists as diverse as: Arthur Capper in the Topeka *Daily Capital*, July 19, 1927, p. 2; Frank Kent in the Baltimore *Sun*, December 10, 1924, p. 1; Paul Y. Anderson in the St. Louis *Post-Dispatch*, October 19, 1925, p. 1; James O'Donnell Bennett in *Liberty* magazine, May 22, 1926; and Richard V. Oulahan, "Hoover, the Handy, Plays Many Parts," *New York Times Magazine*, (November 22, 1925), pp. 3, 16. Writers within the official Hoover circle—Wilhelm, Hunt, Irwin, Sullivan, et al.,—had long been discussing Hoover in such terms.

27. " 'The Master of Emergencies' Film," and A. H. Sawtelle to Lawrence Richey, March 19, 1929, White House Secretaries Files—Lawrence Richey, Presidential Papers, HHP, HHPL.

28. Quoted by Arthur Krock in "President Hoover's Two Years," p. 488; Merlo J. Pusey, *Charles Evans Hughes*, 1:629-30. In a study of Hoover's public image in 1928, Kent M. Schofield has found that magazine and newspaper comment on Hoover's "engineering and administrative" attributes was far wider than discussion of his "humanitarianism" (Kent M. Schofield, "The Figure of Herbert Hoover in the 1928 Campaign" [University of California, Riverside: Ph.D. dissertation, 1966]).

29. It should be noted, however, that two of Hoover's writer friends, Harold Phelps Stokes, his former press secretary, and William Hard had been disturbed by the growth of his image as "an efficiency man, a super expert." Both men felt it was a false image (Harold Phelps Stokes, "Smith and Hoover: A Comparison," p. 1; William Hard, "The New Hoover").

30. Hoover, Public Statements, 60 and 303, HHPL.

31. Mrs. J. H. Flourney to Hoover, August 26, 1922, Hoover to Flourney, August 26, 1922, William Mullendore to Flourney, February 12, 1923, Secretary of Commerce Personal Files, "Flourney"; Hoover to William T. Harris, December 18, 1922, and June 10, 1926, SCOF, "Senate"; Hoover to John Corbin, November 17, 1922, Hoover to R. J. Cuddihy, editor of *Literary Digest*, December 20, 1922, SCPF, "Corbin," "Cuddihy," HHP, HHPL.

32. P. 69. *American Individualism*, though widely distributed by Hoover's aides, such as George Barr Baker, among his many friends and former CRB, Food Administration, and ARA subordinates, never had a wide public reading. Its sentiments, though later expressed by Hoover in his speeches as secretary of commerce and as a presidential candidate, did not alter his public image as a dynamic "social engineer." Perhaps this was due in part to Hoover's refusal to permit "personal

publicity." In any case, detached writers like Walter Millis, confused by Hoover's failure to perform in the White House as advertised, were reading *American Individualism* for the first time and discovering the "real" Hoover (Walter Millis, "The President," pp. 271-73).

33. Ray T. Tucker, "Is Hoover Human?," p. 513.

34. Willis J. Abbot had served under Hoover during his brief editorship of the Washington *Herald* and was a warm supporter of him as editor of the *Christian Science Monitor* (Willis J. Abbot, *Watching the World Go By*, p. 345). Senator George Moses of New Hampshire remembered Hoover as having said, "I have been absurdly over-sold. No man can live up to it" (George Moses as told to George Sylvester Viereck, "The Misunderstood Hoover," *Liberty* [September, 1932]).

35. See Charles Michelson's autobiographical account, *The Ghost Talks*, pp. 15-35.

36. Walter Lippmann, "The Peculiar Weakness of Mr. Hoover," pp. 1-3.

37. Elliott Thurston, "Hoover Can Not Be Elected," pp. 13-14.

38. Fred Fuller Shedd to Verne Marshall, editor of the Cedar Rapids (Iowa) *Evening Gazette*, May 20, 1930, Presidential Papers Official File, HHP, HHPL. Marshall sent copies of Shedd's letter and his own reply on to George Akerson at the White House.

39. Paul Y. Anderson, "Hoover and the Press."

40. An anonymous reporter in discussing Hoover's White House staff—George Akerson, Lawrence Richey, French Strother, and Walter Newton—wrote, for instance: "It was to be expected that the appearance in the White House of a Big Executive should see [the] massing of secretarial help. In bygone days the President had *a* secretary. . . . But that was before the era of the Super-Administrator, before Efficiency came to the White House" (A Washington Correspondent, "The Secretariat," p. 385). In a recent interview, Robert S. Allen has revealed himself as the writer of this article (Robert Allen interviewed by Raymond Henle, director, Herbert Hoover Oral History Program, November 11, 1966, p. 2, HHPL).

41. See above, note 33; below, note 48.

42. [Ray Thomas Tucker], *The Mirrors of 1932*, pp. 1-30.

43. Robert Herrick, "Our Super-Babbitt: A Recantation," p. 60.

43. Heywood Broun, "It Seems to Heywood Broun."

45. [Robert Allen and Drew Pearson], *Washington Merry-Go-Round*, p. 77; see also, Allen, *Why Hoover Faces Defeat*, pp. 1-37.

46. Hoover, *State Papers*, I, Public Statement, 2, "Relations of the President with the Press: Remarks Made at First Press Conference," March 5, 1929, pp. 12-13; George Akerson to Robert Barry, November 4, 1930, with enclosed memorandum describing Hoover's press relations, George E. Akerson Papers, HHPL.

47. Memorandum, Mark Sullivan [to Hoover], "Press Conferences," March, 1929, Presidential Papers White House Secretarial Files—Lawrence Richey Files, HHP, HHPL.

48. George H. Manning, "Hoover Liberalizes Press Conferences: New Chief Executive Expected to Take Correspondents into Confidence," p. 7; Ray T. Tucker, "Mr. Hoover Lays a Ghost," pp. 662-69.

49. See, for instance, Hoover to Walter Lippmann, September 30, 1924, Hoover to Fred Essary, April 27, 1925, and Hoover to editors and correspondents of the Baltimore *Sun*, April 21, 1926, SCPF, "Newspapers"; Hoover to Richard H. Edmonds, October 11, 1924, SCPF, "Edmunds," HHP, HHPL. The writers were not

the only people who occasionally pricked Hoover's "thin-skin." A staunch defender of the prerogatives he had established in accepting the position of secretary of commerce, Hoover also let his fellow cabinet members feel the sting of his anger when he believed they were encroaching on these prerogatives (Hoover to Secretary of State Charles Evans Hughes, December 15, 1921, SCPF, "Hughes, Charles Evans"; Hoover to Secretary of Labor James J. Davis, April 15, 1924, SCOF, "Twelve-Hour Day"; Hoover to Hughes, February 28, 1925, SCOF, "Commerce Department Foreign and Domestic Commerce, Miscellaneous," HHP, HHPL). The secretary's sense of the superiority of his own department over the others was manifested in a letter to an Ohio congressman requesting that he recommend a man for the department's solicitor position. "While the other Departments can get along with a man who knows the law," he wrote, "I have got to have somebody who has a large vision of public affairs, the business world, etc." (Hoover to James T. Begg, June 22, 1927, SCOF, "House of Representatives," HHP, HHPL).

50. Within two weeks of taking office, Hoover had fired his initial director of the Bureau of Foreign and Domestic Commerce, R. S. MacElwee, for giving information to the press without his permission. A month later, bothered by "misstatements of facts" coming out of his press conferences, he had called upon the newsmen to organize a special committee within their ranks "to control 'breaks' " and "also violations of confidence." Two years later, he required all statements of his subordinates in the department "implying economic interpretation, forecasting, or advice," to be sent to his office for his personal approval "before going to the Mimeograph Room or to the printer." This order briefly raised the charge of censorship (SCOF, "Commerce, Foreign and Domestic Commerce, Bureau of, MacElwee, Roy S."; Memorandum Croghan to Herter, April 18, 1921, Confidential Memorandum Hoover to Croghan, April 23, 1923, William L. Daley, United Publishers Corporation, to Hoover, May 28, 1923, SCOF, "Commerce, Foreign and Domestic, Bureau of, Croghan, 1921-25," HHP, HHPL).

51. Bess Furman, *Washington By-Line: The Personal History of a Newspaper Woman,* pp. 6-9.

52. Baker's stated reason for his close supervision of the dispatches was merely to expedite the sending process and to "avoid confusion." His actions were "not a censorship" (Memorandum, Baker to Lieutenant Mather, at sea en route to Rio de Janeiro, December 18, 1928, Campaign and Pre-Inaugural Papers, 1928-1929, HHP, HHPL). An editorial in the Baltimore *Sun,* however, characterized Baker's dispatch policy as "insufferable" and averred that what was at issue was not the length of the dispatches, but their contents (quoted in "Censorship on Mr. Hoover's Trip?," *Army and Navy Register* 85 [January 19, 1929]: 59).

53. George H. Manning, " 'Tightening' of Press Relations Irks Washington Correspondents," p. 25. Hoover had once tried to arrange the firing of a reporter who had merely speculated about his political plans. He felt the writer represented the "interest" of California Senator Hiram Johnson, a man whose bid for the Republican nomination in 1920 he had purposefully spoiled with his own entry into the California primary (Hoover, *Memoirs,* 2:34-35). In 1925, Hoover wired his political informant in California, Mark Requa: "I refer you to article by McClatchey appearing in Oakland *Tribune* of September 20th headed Presidency for Hoover. Same appears San Francisco *Bulletin.* This fellow engaged all times in opposition and intrigue against myself and these articles are intended to make jealousies and trouble here. Will you see Holman and Knowland and see if you cannot get dismissed and some man appointed as their correspondent who does not represent Johnson interest" (Hoover to Mark Requa, October 5, 1925, SCPF, "Requa, M. L., 1925-1928," HHP, HHPL). Lest one assume that this great sensitivity to specula-

tion about his political motives suggests that Hoover harbored "secret" political ambitions, it should be noted that even as president he reacted almost as bitterly when newsmen, in his words, "ascribed personal and partisan political" motives to his speaking tour of the Middle West in 1931 (Hoover to Roy Howard, Scripps-Howard Newspapers, June 22, 1931, Presidential Papers Official File, HHP, HHPL). What seems to have been at stake in his attempt to have McClatchey fired was his strong need to be regarded as nonpartisan, not a deep-seated political ambition. The latter, in my opinion, never existed.

54. A Washington Correspondent, "The Secretariat," p. 393; Anderson, "Hoover and the Press," p. 383.

55. Manning, " 'Tightening' of Press Relations Irks Washington Correspondents," p. 25.

56. Manning, "White House Is Best News Source for Rapidan Camp 100 Miles Away," p. 15.

57. Harold Brayman, "Hooverizing the Press"; John S. Gregory, "All Quiet on the Rapidan," pp. 427-28.

58. Akerson to Robert Barry, Memorandum on Hoover's press relations, November 4, 1930, Akerson Papers, HHPL; Theodore Joslin, *Hoover off the Record*, p. 69; Hoover to Byron Price, Associated Press, May 2, 1931, Presidential Papers President's Personal File, HHP, HHPL; Richey, who ever since the Food Administration period had served Hoover as an investigator of press "leaks" and, as Bradley Nash has put it, as a "protector of his privacy," was very active in this capacity during Hoover's presidency. In addition to ferreting out the sources of "leaks," he investigated and maintained a "black list" of those individuals who, writing anonymously, had turned against the president (Lewis L. Strauss to Richey, October 17 and October 25, 1932, Presidential Papers White House Secretaries Files—Lawrence Richey Files; French Strother to Richey, September 12, 1932, White House Secretaries Files—French Strother Files, HHP, HHPL; Bradley Nash interviewed by Raymond Henle, Director, Herbert Hoover Oral History Program, July 31, 1968, pp. 3-4, HHPL).

59. A Washington Correspondent, "The Secretariat," pp. 392-94; Anderson, "A Cross-Section of Washington," p. 420; Brayman, "Hooverizing the Press," pp. 123-24; Gregory, "All Quiet on the Rapidan," pp. 427-28; Anderson, "Hoover and the Press," pp. 382-84; [Pearson and Allen], *Washington Merry-Go-Round*, pp. 51-77, 302-50; Allen, *Why Hoover Faces Defeat*, pp. 89-92.

60. Karl A. Bickle to Tom Gregory, July 8, 1929, Gregory to Akerson, July 31, 1929, Akerson Papers, HHPL.

61. Akerson to Gregory, August 6, 1929, Akerson Papers, HHPL.

62. A. W. Kirchhofer to Hoover, July 18, 1930, Presidential Papers President's Personal File, HHP, HHPL.

63. Ibid.

64. Hoover to Kirchhofer, July 18, 1930, Presidential Papers President's Personal File, HHP, HHPL. Fifteen months later, Kirchhofer was repeating much the same mixture of criticism and advice, prefacing his remarks with the comment: "I shouldn't be telling such a veteran as you are in dealing with the press what the fundamentals of that game are. So I simply set them down as a reminder" (Kirchhofer to Hoover, September 1, 1931, Presidential Papers White House Secretaries Files—Lawrence Richey Files, HHP, HHPL).

65. Joslin, *Hoover off the Record*, pp. 12-24.

66. Ibid., pp. 4, 69-71.

67. Hoover's steps to supervise closely all news passing out of the Department of Commerce had also been motivated by his desire to maintain "psychological confidence" in the economy.

68. Evidently this strategy was now backfiring. A standard joke making the rounds in Washington observed that every time the president released an optimistic statement, the stockmarket dropped even lower (see [Allen and Pearson], *Washington Merry-Go-Round*, p. 61). If Charles Michelson's account is to be believed, Hoover actually instigated an investigation of Michelson's employer, John J. Rascob, the Democratic party national chairman, in a futile effort to prove that Rascob had been using his weight on Wall Street to produce just such an effect (Michelson, *The Ghost Talks*, pp. 25-26).

69. Hoover was the first American president to have a telephone installed in his office. In the fall of 1931, Walter Lippmann was observing that "scarcely a week passes but some new story comes out of Washington as to how Mr. Hoover has had somebody on the telephone and is attempting to fix this situation or that" (Lippmann, *Interpretations, 1931-1932*, ed. Allan Nevins, p. 68).

70. Hoover to Arthur T. Robb, managing editor, *Editor and Publisher*, April 4, 1930; Hoover to Harry Chandler, November 3, 1931, Presidential Papers President's Personal File, HHP, HHPL.

71. Kent Cooper, *Kent Cooper and the Associated Press: An Autobiography*, pp. 156-57; Isaac F. Marcosson, *Before I Forget: A Pilgrimage to the Past*, pp. 458-59.

72. A detailed account of the progressive deterioration of Hoover's presidential press relations—an account drawn largely from George Manning's many reports in *Editor and Publisher*—may be found in James E. Pollard, *The Presidents and the Press*, pp. 737-72

73. Woods to Akerson, November 25, 1930, Presidential Papers Official File, HHP, HHPL; Abbot, *Watching the World Go By*, p. 345; William Hard to French Strother, n.d., Presidential Papers White House Secretaries Files—French Strother Files; William Allen White to David Hinshaw, July 9, 1932, Presidential Papers White House Secretaries Files—Lawrence Richey Files, HHP, HHPL; David Lawrence interviewed by Raymond Henle, director, Herbert Hoover Oral History Program, February 8, 1968, p. 18, HHPL.

74. See Erwin Knoll's article, "The President and the Press: Eliminating the Middlemen," in which he observes that ever since his famous "Checkers speech," Nixon has used the effective strategy of "talk[ing] over the heads of the press to the people."

75. See the sympathetic criticisms of Hoover's public speaking in Henry F. Pringle, "Hoover: An Enigma Easily Misunderstood," p. 131; in Iowa Congressman Cyrenus Cole's memoirs, *I Remember, I Remember: A Book of Recollections*, pp. 402-3; and Joslin, *Hoover off the Record*, p. 7.

76. Edmund W. Starling, a Secret Service man in Hoover's entourage, has recalled that he devised a special elevated reading stand to lift the president's face and thus improve the affect of his public appearances. Still, he remained "a poor speaker" (E. W. Starling, *Starling of the White House*, pp. 285-86); Elmer Cornwell, *Presidential Leadership of Public Opinion*, pp. 112-13; Hoover was evidently painfully aware of his inability to inspire, for he once asked Bruce Barton to "suggest a line" for a speech "that would be helpful and inspiring" (Hoover to Barton, May 16, 1930, Presidential Papers President's Personal File, HHP, HHPL). In congratulating George Lorimer on a moving editorial in the *Saturday Evening Post* about the affects of the depression on the country, Hoover remarked: "I regret that I do

not possess your quality of expressions although I have feelings that probably are as deep as your own" (Hoover to Lorimer, May 31, 1931, Presidential Papers President's Personal File, HHP, HHPL).

77. Quoted in Eugene Lyons, *Our Unknown Ex-President: A Portrait of Herbert Hoover*, p. 27; Joslin, *Hoover off the Record*, p. 3.

78. As early as December, 1930, Hoover had requested A. H. Kirchhofer to start preparing a "publicity scheme" for the 1932 campaign (Kirchhofer to Hoover, January 8, 1931, Hoover to Kirchhofer, January 13, 1931, Presidential Papers President's Personal File, HHP, HHPL).

79. Though habitually geared to the guidance of public opinion, Hoover, at times of heated public controversy or when under personal attack, had in the past tended to withdraw from debating the issue. For instance, he had decided not to speak out against federal repression during the "Red Scare" of 1920, for given the "generally reactionary atmosphere" it was "better to await [a] more favorable turn of public opinion before trying to secure reason" (Hoover to Ray Lyman Wilbur, April 17, 1920, Pre-Commerce, "1920 Campaign," HHP, HHPL). When asked by a friend to resume his once strong advocacy for the League of Nations, he had replied: "There are times in public sentiment when it is utterly impossible to make a dent and . . . we are in one of those periods now so far as the American people are concerned" (Hoover to Frederick R. Coudert, August 25, 1922, SCPF, "Coudert," HHP, HHPL). As for replying to personal attacks, Hoover's attitude had often been that "every man in the street knows the futility of trying to overtake a misrepresentation once made" (Hoover to Richard Edmonds, October 11, 1924, SCPF, "Edmonds," HHP, HHPL). When urged as president to respond to Michelson's charges and the "smear" books, his response was much the same: "No man can catch up with a lie. If the American people wish to believe such things as this about me, it just cannot be helped" (quoted in Joslin, *Hoover off the Record*, p. 37).

80. Akerson, "A Day with the President," Radio Address; Akerson to Alan Fox, June 12, 1930, Akerson Papers, HHPL. The "problem of humanizing" went back before the trying times of the depression to the 1928 campaign. Republican publicity director, Henry Allen, had been reported as saying at that time: "You know we've had a lot of trouble with our candidate. Some moron said the thing we've got to do with Hoover is humanize him. We've not been able to do much with him. . . . He wouldn't have his picture taken with a mule to the humanization of both" (quoted in Furman, *Washington By-Line*, pp. 9-10).

81. Joslin, *Hoover off the Record*, pp. 9-11, 80-81; *Time*, 17 (April 27, 1931): 13; Silas Bent, "The Humanizing of Hoover," pp. 288-90; J. Frederick Essary, "Uncle Sam's Ballyhoo Men," pp. 427-28.

82. Will Irwin, "Herbert Hoover: An Intimate Portrait"; Irwin, "These Whispers about Mr. Hoover"; Vernon Kellogg, "The President as I Know Him"; Robert P. Lamont, "The Personality of President Hoover." (The manuscript for this article, prepared by Strother, is found in Presidential Papers White House Secretaries Files —French Strother, HHP, HHPL).

83. Anderson, "A Cross Section of Washington," p. 419; Brayman, "Hooverizing the Press," p. 124; Anderson, "Food and Drink in Washington"; Silas Bent, "Mr. Hoover's Sins of Commissions," pp. 9-10; Essary, "Uncle Sam's Ballyhoo Men," p. 428; [Allen and Pearson], *Washington Merry-Go-Round*, p. 316.

84. David Hinshaw to Hoover, September 28, 1930, Presidential Papers President's Personal File, HHP, HHPL.

85. Typewritten manuscript for *Washington*, "The Handicaps of Hoover,"

Presidential Papers White House Secretaries Files—French Strother Files, HHP, HHPL.

86. Newspaper clipping containing article by Frederick Wile, " 'Washington's,' G.O.P. Paper Survives Only Three Editions," December 4, 1930, Presidential Papers White House Secretaries Files—French Strother Files, HHP, HHPL.

87. Bennett Gordon to Baker, September 5, 1930, George Barr Baker Papers, Box 12, "Republican Clubs, 1924-1932," Hoover Institution on War, Revolution, and Peace.

88. Baker to Robert H. Lucas, December 18, 1931; Rickard to Lucas, December 19, 1931, George Barr Baker Papers, Box 4, "Lucas, Robert H.," Hoover Institution on War, Revolution, and Peace.

89. Kirchhofer to Hoover, July 18, 1930, Presidential Papers President's Personal File, HHP, HHPL. Michelson's basic publicity tactic was to "plant" interviews, statements, and speeches with prominent Democratic members of the House and Senate whose utterances were certain to be picked up by newsmen and editors (Michelson, *The Ghost Talks*, p. 32). Such a tactic was especially effective when contrasted to the administration practice, now increasingly suspect among the press corps, of issuing "handouts" through press agents. Even Frank Kent, a pro-Hoover journalist whose "exposé" of Michelson was reprinted and distributed in summary form by the Republican National Committee in the fall of 1930, admitted: "[Michelson's performance] has been—and still is—a remarkable [one], an illuminating illustration of the amazing power of unopposed propaganda in skillful hands. . . . Mr. Michelson is a man of high intelligence and unquestioned character, a combination so rarely found on a party pay-roll as to be practically non-existent." These admissions, of course, were omitted in the Republican reprint of the article (Frank Kent, "Charley Michelson," pp. 290, 293; Republican National Committee pamphlet, "Democratic Journalist Discloses Real Purpose of Publicity Bureau," (September, 1930), Akerson Papers, HHPL).

90. Kirchhofer to Hoover, September 1, 1931, Presidential Papers White House Secretaries Files—Lawrence Richey Files, HHP, HHPL.

91. Ibid.

92. Republican National Committee Memorandum, October 2, 1932, Presidential Papers Official File, HHP, HHPL.

93. Roy V. Peel, *The 1932 Campaign: An Analysis*, p. 56.

94. See, for instance, William Hard, "Hoover as Individualist"; Bruce Barton, "Shall I Vote for Hoover." Barton's answer was a reluctant "yes"; William Allen White to M. F. Amrine, February 4, 1931, and White to Theodore Roosevelt, Febuary 1, 1933, in Walter Johnson, ed., *The Selected Letters of William Allen White, 1899-1943*, pp. 311, 329.

95. Quoted in Joslin, *Hoover off the Record*, p. 11.

Conclusion

GIVEN THE PAUCITY of primary research materials, historical writing on Herbert Hoover has hitherto tended to dwell understandably on Hoover the businessman, the engineer, and the administrator. In this book, an attempt has been made to highlight an aspect of the man that was just as significant as these, namely Hoover the editorializer, the mobilizer of the press, and the instigator of public relations campaigns. Throughout his public career, he worked from behind the scenes through figureheads, committees, conferences, and the printed media to gain an "outside" influence over men and events. Desirous of holding leverage over public affairs but temperamentally unsuited by shyness and sensitivity for the demands of political life, he contemplated newspaper management and editorial influence as early as 1914 and actually did purchase shares in several papers in 1919 and 1920. Then, after chance and circumstance had conspired to arrange his long sought-after entry into public life, he accommodated the requirements of his personality by becoming a kind of administrative editorialist, relying heavily on the press and public relations to "reach out to the public" and thus to gain support for his policies and programs in the years from 1914 to 1928.

To assist famine-threatened Belgium, he used techniques that he had "rehearsed" in London as a lobbyist for the Panama-Pacific Exposition and proceeded to wield the "club of public opinion" through press campaigns, press agents, committee-organization, and public relations aides. As the American food and relief administrator, he used similar techniques and personnel to "educate and direct public opinion" on the need for food conservation and the postwar reconstruction of Europe. And as secretary of commerce, public relations figured heavily and essentially in his efforts to "stimulate the community to action" in support of his program for American economic development.

In addition, although developed primarily to suit his personality needs, Hoover's dependence upon a behind-the-scenes, public relations style of administration was reinforced in the postwar years by his desire as a progressive to resolve the tension between his elitist reliance upon experts and his commitment to the democratic ethos. For him, in other words, publicity became a means by which to bridge the gap between the experts, who provided social and economic guidelines, and the citizens who executed them. It was for this purpose, not the frequently alleged one of clearing a path to the White House, that he employed numerous press and public relations aides. Yet in practice and despite his constant warnings against "personal publicity," his public relations style did produce an image of him as an economic and engineering mastermind for American society; and this, coupled with the "grass roots" contacts that such an approach developed, eventually culminated in an unstoppable "Hoover boom" for the presidency in 1928.

As president, though, Hoover's idiosyncratic administrative *modus operandi* proved disastrous against the background of the Great Depression. The country required and expected forceful personal leadership and decisive federal initiatives, but Hoover, a prisoner of past administrative habit and growing political and moral convictions, could not provide these. As the depression deepened and he, in response, retreated farther and farther into the background, the compound of personal qualities and administrative procedures that had once seemed so successful and had so impressed the public and the press began to produce hostility and the stereotype of a thoroughly incompetent, heartless, and reactionary figure—a stereotype that has never fully been erased from the American mind. In reality, the circumstances and problems had changed, not the man or his style. On the contrary, his presidential activities were fully in keeping with his lifelong approach to administration, and his postpresidential activities would reflect the same blend of aggresson and introversion.

"I can say that never in the last fifteen years have I had the peace of mind that I have had since the election. I have almost a feeling of elation. My only concern is what will happen to the country as a result of the change in policies."[1] Thus, Hoover summed up his attitudes toward his defeat. Though the interregnum months between the election and the inauguration of his successor were troubled by the banking crisis, which forced him to continue his incredibly long working hours in the White House, from a personal standpoint, they were perhaps the most pleasant of his presidency. Unchallenged now by impossible standards and unbothered by office-seekers and his intrusive enemies in the press, he found some time to relax with his friends and give thought to his future. He did not plan to make any final statement as president, for the "air," as he put it, was already too "full of his words" from the campaign. Though Washington speculated about his plans for a "comeback," he foresaw nothing more than "getting out of the picture" as had always been his wont. For awhile, at least, he desired only to be "a very private citizen."[2]

For two years after he left the White House, Hoover remained "behind the wall of silence" that Joslin admitted he had thrown up around his presidency.[3] Amused, yet also concerned by the "Roosevelt hysteria" in the press and by what George Akerson called "the publicity madness of the whole [Roosevelt] family,"[4] he refused to sanction attacks on Roosevelt or to publish any statements of his own. In early 1934, he wrote Akerson that he disapproved of the impending publication of Joslin's *Hoover off the Record*, for, "whatever the book may be," Joslin would not "have an audience for a long time yet—and you know my feeling about personal publicity."[5]

However, increasingly disturbed by Roosevelt's policies, Hoover, within a year, had changed his mind and decided to break his silence. As he had once planned to do in 1914 and again in 1920, he now finally embarked upon the career of "outside editorial influence"; and reverting to his pre-presidential style, he renewed his old association with Ben Allen and sought the assistance of other journalists in order to "promulgate his ideas" on the "American system" and to "crusade against the New Deal."[6] His reason for taking up residence in New York City, where he would spend

much of his later life, is very revealing of the concern for public
relations that had underlain his whole life in administration:

> New York is the place from where a large part of America's in-
> tellectual life is transmitted. Here centers the control of much
> of the magazine, the book, and the radio world. Some of its daily
> papers spread into every other newspaper office in the coun-
> try. The control of many national charitable and educational in-
> stitutions is centered here because of the closeness to "big
> money." A multitude of political, social, economic, and propa-
> ganda organizations spread out to infiltrate into the whole of
> American life from this great city. When one is interested also
> in the promulgation of ideas, it is more effective to be at the dis-
> tributing point than at the receiving end.[7]

In 1934, in a new city and under new social and economic conditions, Herbert Hoover resumed the career, so congenial to his
personality and philosophy, which he had abandoned for the crush-
ing burdens of the presidency.

1.   Theodore Joslin, *Hoover off the Record*, p. 328.

2.   Anne O'Hare McCormick, "Hoover Looks Back—and Ahead," *New York Times Magazine*, February 5, 1933, p. 1.

3.   Joslin, *Hoover off the Record*, p. 367.

4.   George E. Akerson to Hoover, March 23, 1933; Hoover to Akerson, March 27, 1933, George E. Akerson Papers, HHPL.

5.   Hoover to Akerson, January 9, 1934, Akerson Papers, HHPL.

6.   Ben S. Allen File, Herbert Hoover Archives, Hoover Institution on War, Revolution, and Peace. *Time* linked Hoover's reemergence as a public commentator in 1935 to the return of Allen as his "adviser, contactman, and traveling companion" ("Political Notes: Presidential Prose," *Time* 26 [December 30, 1934]: 8); Paul C. Smith, *Personal File* (New York, 1964), pp. 157-59; Herbert Hoover, *The Memoirs of Herbert Hoover: The Great Depression, 1929-1941* (New York, 1952), 3:346-47.

7.   Ibid.

Bibliography

Manuscript Collections

Herbert Hoover Presidential Library
  Herbert Hoover Papers
    Pre-Commerce Papers
    Commerce Papers
    Presidential Papers
  George E. Akerson Papers
  Ben Allen Papers
  Frederick M. Feiker Papers
Hoover Institution on War, Revolution, and Peace
  American Relief Administration Papers
  Food Administration Files
  George Barr Baker Papers
  Hugh Gibson Collection
  Edward Eyre Hunt Collection
  Mark Sullivan Collection
  Ray Lyman Wilbur Papers

Public Documents

Conference on Unemployment, Washington, D.C., 1921. *Report of the President's Conference on Unemployment*. Washington: Government Printing Office, 1921.

Hoover, Herbert. "Foreword." *Seasonal Operation in the Construction Industries: Summary of Report and Recommendations*. Committee of the President's Conference on Unemployment, 1921. Washington: Government Printing Office, 1924.

———. "Introduction." United States Department of Commerce. *Trade Association Activities*. Washington, D.C., Government Printing Office, 1923.

United States. Department of Commerce. *Annual Report of the Secretary of Commerce*, Ninth-Fourteenth, 1921-26. Washington: Government Printing Office, 1921-26.

United States. Department of Commerce. *Simplified Practice: What It Is and What It Offers*. Issued by the Bureau of Standards, November 26, 1924. Washington: Government Printing Office, 1924.

Books

Abbot, Willis J. *Watching the World Go by*. Boston: Little, Brown & Co., 1933.

Allen, Robert S. *Why Hoover Faces Defeat*. New York: Bohn & Co., 1932.

[Allen, Robert S., and Drew Pearson]. *Washington Merry-Go-Round*. New York: Liveright, Inc., 1932.

Angell, Norman. *After All: The Autobiography of Norman Angell*. New York: Farrar, Straus, & Young, 1951.

———. *The Great Illusion: A Study of the Relation of Military Power to Their Economic and Social Advantage*. New York: George P. Putnam's Sons, 1910.

Austin, Mary. *Earth Horizon: Autobiography*. Boston: Houghton Mifflin Co., 1932.

Bernays, Edward L. *Biography of an Idea: Memoirs of Public Relations Counsel Edward L. Bernays*. New York: Simon & Schuster, 1965.

Bernstein, Barton J. "The New Deal: The Conservative Achievements of Liberal Reform," in *Towards a New Past: Dissenting Essays in American History*. Edited by Barton J. Bernstein. New York, Pantheon Books, 1968.

Blainey, Geoffrey. *The Rush That Never Ended: A History of Australian Mining*. Melbourne: Melbourne University Press, 1963.

Bok, Edward W. *Twice Thirty*. New York: Charles Scribner's Sons, 1925.

Brandes, Joseph. *Herbert Hoover and Economic Diplomacy: Department of Commerce Policy, 1921-1928*. Pittsburgh: University of Pittsburgh Press, 1962.

Britt, George. *Forty Years—Forty Millions: The Career of Frank A. Munsey*. New York: Farrar & Rinehart, Inc., 1935.

Cole, Cyrenus. *I Remember, I Remember: A Book of Recollections*. Iowa City, Iowa: State Historical Society of Iowa, 1936.

Cooper, Kent. *Kent Cooper and the Associated Press: An Autobiography*. New York: Random House, 1959.

Copeland, Melvin T. *And Mark an Era: The Story of the Harvard Business School*. Boston: Little, Brown, 1958.

Corey, Herbert. *The Truth about Hoover*. Boston: Houghton Mifflin Co., 1932.

Cornwell, Elmer E., Jr. *Presidential Leadership of Public Opinion*. Bloomington, Ind.: Indiana University Press, 1965.

Creel, George. *How We Advertised America*. New York: Harper & Bros., 1920.

Dangerfield, George. *The Strange Death of Liberal England, 1910-1914*. New York: Harrison Smith & Robert Hass, Inc., 1935.

Daniels, Josephus. *The Wilson Era: Years of War and After, 1917-1923*. Chapel Hill: University of North Carolina, 1946.

De Conde, Alexander. *A History of American Foreign Policy*. New York: Charles Scribner's Sons, 1963.

Furman, Bess. *Washington By-Line: The Personal History of a Newspaper Woman*. New York: Alfred A. Knopf, 1949.

Galambos, Louis. *Competition and Cooperation: The Emergence of a National Trade Association*. Baltimore: Johns Hopkins Press, 1966.

Gay, George I., with the collaboration of H. H. Fisher, *Public Relations of the Commission for Relief in Belgium: Documents*. 2 vols. Stanford, Calif.: Stanford University Press, 1929.

[Gilbert, Clinton W.] *The Mirrors of Washington*. New York: George P. Putnam's Sons, 1921.

Goldman, Eric Frederick. *Two-Way Street: The Emergence of the Public Relations Counsel*. Boston: Bellman Publishing Co., 1948.

Graham, Otis L., Jr. *An Encore for Reform: The Old Progressives and the New Deal*. New York: Oxford University Press, 1967.

Guerrier, Edith. *We Pledged Allegiance: A Librarian's Intimate Story of the United States Food Administration*. Stanford, Calif.: Stanford University Press, 1941.

Haber, Samuel. *Efficiency and Uplift: Scientific Management in the Progressive Era, 1890-1920*. Chicago: University of Chicago Press, 1964.

Hard, William. *Who's Hoover?* New York: Dodd, Mead & Co., 1928.

Heaton, Herbert. *A Scholar in Action: Edwin F. Gay*. Cambridge: Harvard University Press, 1952.

Hicks, John D. *Republican Ascendancy, 1921-1933*. New York: Harper & Bros., 1960.

Hinshaw, David. *Herbert Hoover: American Quaker*. New York: Farrar, Straus & Co., 1950.

Hofstadter, Richard. *The Age of Reform: From Bryan to F.D.R.* New York: Alfred A. Knopf, 1955.

——. *The American Political Tradition and the Men Who Made It*. New York: Alfred A. Knopf, Inc., 1948.

Hoover, Herbert. *An American Epic*. 4 vols. Chicago: Regnery Co., 1959-60.

——. *American Individualism*. Garden City, N.Y.: Doubleday, Page & Co., 1922.

——. "Foreword," in *America and the New Era: A Symposium on Social Reconstruction*. Edited by Elisha M. Friedman. New York: E. P. Dutton & Co., 1920.

——. "Foreword," *Unemployment and Business Cycles*. New York: McGraw-Hill Book Co., Inc., 1923.

——. "Foreword," *Waste in Industry*. New York: McGraw Hill Book Co., Inc., 1921.

——. "Introduction," *The Stabilization of Business*. Edited by Lionel D. Edie. New York: Macmillan Co., 1923.

——. *The Memoirs of Herbert Hoover*. 3 vols. New York: Macmillan Co., 1951-52.

——. *The New Day: Campaign Speeches of Herbert Hoover, 1928*. Stanford, Calif.: Stanford University Press, 1928.

——. *Principles of Mining*. New York: Hill Publishing Co., 1909.

——. *The State Papers and Other Public Writings of Herbert Hoover*. Collected and edited by William Starr Meyers. 2 vols. Garden City, N.Y.: Doubleday, Doran & Co., Inc., 1934.

Hunt, Edward Eyre, ed. *Scientific Management Since Taylor: A Collection of Authoritative Papers*. New York: McGraw-Hill Book Co., Inc., 1924.

Irwin, Will. *Herbert Hoover: A Reminiscent Biography*. New York: Century Co., 1928.

——. *The Making of a Reporter*. New York: G. P. Putnam's Sons, 1942.

Jones, Louis Thomas. *The Quakers of Iowa*. Iowa City, Iowa: State Historical Society of Iowa, 1914.

Jordon, David Starr. *The Days of a Man*. 2 vols. Yonkers-on-Hudson, N.Y.: World Book Co., 1922.

Joslin, Theodore G. *Hoover off the Record*. Garden City, N.Y.: Doubleday, Doran & Co., Inc., 1934.

Kellogg, Vernon. *Herbert Hoover: The Man and His Work*. New York: Daniel Appleton & Co., 1920.

Lippmann, Walter. *Interpretations, 1931-1932*. Edited by Allan Nevins. New York: Macmillan Co., 1932.

Lyons, Eugene. *Our Unknown Ex-President: A Portrait of Herbert Hoover*. New York: Doubleday & Co., Inc., 1948.

Marcosson, Isaac F. *Before I Forget: A Pilgrimage to the Past*. New York: Dodd, Mead, 1959.

———. *Caravans of Commerce*. New York: Harper & Bros., 1926.

Mason, Alpheus Thomas. *Brandeis: A Free Man's Life*. New York: Viking Press, 1946.

May, Henry F. *The End of American Innocence*. New York: Alfred A. Knopf, 1959.

McCamy, James L. *Government Publicity: Its Practice in Federal Administration*. Chicago: University of Chicago Press, 1939.

Mencken, H. L., ed. *The Sunpapers of Baltimore, 1837-1937*, by Gerald W. Johnson, Frank R. Kent, H. L. Mencken, and Hamilton Owens. New York: Alfred A. Knopf, 1937.

Merritt, Albert N. *War Time Control of Distribution of Foods*. New York: Macmillan Co., 1920.

Michelson, Charles. *The Ghost Talks*. New York: George P. Putnam's Sons, 1944.

Mowry, George Edwin. *The Urban Nation, 1920-1960*. New York: Hill & Wang, 1965.

———. *The California Progressives*. Berkeley: University of California Press, 1951.

———. *The Era of Theodore Roosevelt, 1900-1912*. New York: Harper & Bros., 1958.

Mullendore, William Clinton. *The History of the United States Food Administration, 1917-1918*, with an Introduction by Herbert Hoover. Stanford, Calif.: Stanford University Press, 1941.

Palmer, Frederick. *With My Own Eyes: A Personal Story of Battle Years*. Indianapolis: Bobbs-Merrill Co., 1933.

Peel, Roy V., and Thomas C. Donnelly. *The 1932 Campaign: An Analysis*. New York: Farrar & Rinehart, Inc., 1935.

Pollard, James E. *The Presidents and the Press*. New York: Macmillan Co., 1947.

Pollack, Ivan L. *The Food Administration in Iowa.* 2 vols. Iowa City: State Historical Society of Iowa, 1923.

Pringle, Henry F. *The Life and Times of William H. Taft: A Biography.* 2 vols. New York: Farrar & Rinehart Inc., 1939.

Pusey, Merlo J. *Charles Evans Hughes.* 2 vols. New York: Columbia University Press, 1963.

Redfield, William C. *With Congress and Cabinet.* Garden City, N.Y.: Doubleday, Page & Co., 1924.

Regier, C. C. *The Era of the Muckrakers.* Chapel Hill: University of North Carolina Press, 1932.

Romasco, Albert U. *The Poverty of Abundance: Hoover, the Nation, the Depression.* New York: Oxford University Press, 1965.

Ross, Edward A. *Seventy Years of It: An Autobiography.* New York: D. Appleton—Century Co., Inc., 1936.

Rosten, Leo C. *The Washington Correspondents.* New York: Harcourt, Brace & Co., 1937.

Rothbard, Murray N. *America's Great Depression.* Princeton, N.J.: D. Van Nostrand Co., Inc., 1963.

Schofield, Kent M. "The Figure of Herbert Hoover in the 1928 Campaign," University of California, Riverside: Ph.D. diss., 1966.

Slosson, Preston W. *The Great Crusade and After, 1914-1928.* New York: Macmillan Co., 1937.

Starling, Edmund W. *Starling of the White House.* New York: Simon & Schuster, 1946.

Stein, Herbert. *The Fiscal Revolution in America.* Chicago: University of Chicago Press, 1969.

Strauss, Lewis L. *Men and Decisions.* Garden City, N.Y.: Doubleday & Co., Inc., 1962.

Sullivan, Mark. *The Education of an American.* New York: Doubleday, Doran & Co., Inc., 1938.

——. *Our Times: The Twenties.* Vol. VI. New York: Charles Scribner's Sons, 1935.

Surface, Frank M., and Raymond L. Bland. *American Food in the World War and Reconstruction Period.* Stanford, Calif.: Stanford University Press, 1931.

Tarbell, Ida M. *All in the Day's Work: An Autobiography.* New York: Macmillan Co., 1939.

Todd, Frank Norton. *The Story of the Exposition.* 5 vols. New York: Published for the Panama-Pacific International Exposition Company, by G. P. Putnam's Sons, 1921.

[Tucker, Ray Thomas]. *The Mirrors of 1932*. New York: Brewer, Warren & Putnam, 1931.

Warren, Harris G. *Herbert Hoover and the Great Depression*. New York: Oxford University Press, 1959.

Weinberg, Arthur and Lila, eds. *The Muckrakers, 1902-1912*. New York: Simon & Schuster, 1961.

Welter, Rush. *Popular Education and Democratic Thought in America*. New York: Columbia University Press, 1962.

White, William Allen. *The Autobiography of William Allen White*. New York: Macmillan Co., 1946.

———. *The Selected Letters of William Allen White, 1899-1943*. Edited, with an Introduction, by Walter Johnson. New York: Henry Holt & Co., 1947.

Wilbur, Ray Lyman. *The Memoirs of Ray Lyman Wilbur, 1875-1949*. Stanford, Calif.: Stanford University Press, 1960.

Williams, William Appleman. *The Contours of American History*. Cleveland: World Publishing Co., 1961.

Zieger, Robert H. *Republicans and Labor, 1919-1929*. Lexington: University of Kentucky Press, 1969.

Articles

[Allen, Robert S.] "The Secretariat," *American Mercury* 18 (December, 1929): 385-95.

Anderson, Paul Y. "A Cross-Section of Washington," *Nation* 130 (April 9, 1930): 419-20.

———. "Food and Drink in Washington," *Nation* 132 (February 11, 1931): 150-51.

———. "Hoover and the Press," *Nation* 133 (October 14, 1931): 382-84.

Austin, Mary. "Hoover and Johnson: West Is West," *Nation* 110 (May 15, 1920): 642-44.

Baker, George Barr. "The Great Fat Fight," *Saturday Evening Post* 200 (May 12, 1928): 12-13, 170, 173-74.

———. "The Pope and the 'Lone Crusader.'" *American Magazine* 83 (March, 1917): 16, 117-18, 120.

"Ballyhoover." *Nation* 130 (May 14, 1930): 560.

Barnes, Julius H. "Herbert Hoover: Some Reasons for His Reputation," *Outlook* 124 (April 14, 1920): 642-44.

Barton, Bruce. "Shall I Vote for Hoover?" *Woman's Home Companion* 59 (October, 1932): 9-10, 93-95.

Bent, Silas. "The Humanizing of Hoover," *Scribner's Magazine* 90 (July, 1931): 9-14
——. "Mr. Hoover's Sins of Commissions," *Scribner's Magazine* 90 (July, 1931): 9-14.
Blythe, Samuel. "A Calm Review of a Calm Man," *Saturday Evening Post* 196 (July 28, 1923): 3-4.
Brayman, Harold. "Hooverizing the Press," *Outlook and Independent* 156 (September 24, 1930): 123-25.
Broun, Heywood. "It Seems to Heywood Broun," *Nation* 130 (July 25, 1930): 723.
"Business Editors Will Help Hoover Solve Nation's Trade Problems," *Editor and Publisher* 53 (April 16, 1921): 11.
Cowell, F. R. "Government Departments and the Press in the U.S.A.," *Public Administration* 9 (April, 1931): 214-27.
Degler, Carl. "The Ordeal of Herbert Hoover," *Yale Review* 52 (June, 1963): 563-83.
Dennis, Alfred P. "Humanizing the Department of Commerce," *Saturday Evening Post* 197 (June 6, 1925): 8-9.
Essary, J. Frederick. "Uncle Sam's Ballyhoo Men," *American Mercury* 23 (August, 1931): 419-28.
Feiker, Frederick. "The Profession of Commerce in the Making," *Annals of the American Academy of Political and Social Science* 101 (May, 1922): 203-7.
——. "The Trend of 'Simplification': How the Movement Is Growing and What the Paving Brick Action Signifies," *Factory* 28 (February, 1922): 156-58.
——. "What the Department of Commerce Is Doing for Industry," *Electrical World* 79 (January 14, 1922): 71-73.
George, Alexander L. "Power as a Compensatory Value for Political Leaders," *Journal of Social Issues* 24, No. 3 (July, 1968): 29-49.
Gibson, Hugh S. "Herbert Clark Hoover," *Century* 94 (August, 1917): 508-17.
Gregory, John S. "All Quiet on the Rapidan," *Outlook and Independent* 158 (August 5, 1931): 427, 434-435.
Hard, William. "Hoover as Individualist," *Nation* 133 (August 26, 1931): 201-3.
——. "The New Hoover," *American Review of Reviews* 86 (November, 1927): 478-84.
"Hearst Buys *Herald* in Washington," *Editor and Publisher* 55 (November 18, 1922): 16.

Herrick, Robert. "Our Super-Babbitt: A Recantation," *Nation* 131 (July 16, 1930): 60-62.

Herter, C. A. "Looking Back on Kansas City," *Independent* 120 (June 30, 1928): 614-16.

Holt, Hamilton. "When Mr. Hoover Talks," *Review of Reviews* 78 (December, 1928): 589.

Hoover, Herbert. "America and You," *Open Road* 1 (May, 1920).

——. "Bind the Wounds of France," *National Geographic Magazine* 31 (May, 1917): 439-44.

——. "Conserving the Food Supply," *Engineering and Mining Journal* 104 (July 21, 1917): 125-27.

——. "Economic, Social, and Industrial Problems Confronting the Nation: Maintenance of Our National Ideals," *Trust Companies* 30 (April, 1920): 349-52.

——. "Facing Our Economic Facts," *Columbia* 1 (August, 1921): 3.

——. "Fact Information in Business," *Special Libraries* 12 (April, 1921): 61.

——. "The Food Future: What Every American Mouthful Means to Europe," *Forum* 61 (February, 1919): 210-18.

——. "The Food Situation in Liberated Territories," *Commercial and Financial Chronicle* 108 (January 11, 1919): 118-19.

——. "The Home as an Investment," *Delineator* 101 (October, 1922): 17.

——. "The Housing Problem: A Direct Message for Responsible Industrial Executives," *Industrial Management* 60 (December, 1920): 424a-24b.

——. "A Little Child Shall Lead," *Good Housekeeping* 76 (June, 1923): 27, 118, 121-22, 125-26, 128-29.

——. "Neighborhood (Settlement) Houses Help Solve Social Problems," *Better Times* 1 (June, 1920).

——. "The New Food Card," *Journal of Home Economics* 10 (January, 1918): 21-22.

——. "The Paramount Business of Every American Today," *System* 38 (July, 1920): 23-25.

——. "Self-Expression Is the Need of Today," *Business Methods*, November, 1920.

——. "Some Notes on Industrial Readjustment," *Saturday Evening Post* 192 (December 27, 1919): 3-4, 145-46.

——. "What America Faces," *Industrial Management* 61 (April 1, 1921): 225-29.

Hunt, Edward Eyre. "A Long Step Forward," *Survey* 47 (December 17, 1921): 427-29.

———. "Government and Trade Associations," *Outlook* 130 (March 1, 1922): 352-55.

———. "How Industry Can Avoid Summer Depression," *Printer's Ink* 119 (May 18, 1922): 8-12.

Irwin, Will. "First Aid to America," *Saturday Evening Post* 189 (March 24, 1917): 6-7, 109-10, 113-14.

———. "The First Ward Ball," *Collier's* 42 (February 6, 1909): 16-17.

———. "Herbert Hoover: An Intimate Portrait," *American Magazine* 109 (May, 1930): 16-17, 126.

———. "Hoover as an Executive," *Saturday Evening Post* 192 (March 27, 1920), 5, 70, 73-74, 76, 79.

———. "These Whispers about Mr. Hoover," *Liberty*, May 21, 1932, pp. 11-15.

Jordan, David Starr. "Interesting Westerners," *Sunset* 34 (June, 1915): 1175-79.

Kellogg, Vernon. "Herbert Hoover as Individual and Type," *Atlantic Monthly* 121 (March, 1918): 375-85.

———. "The President As I Know Him," *Atlantic Monthly* 150 (July, 1932): 1-12.

———. "Washington Five and Eight O'Clocks," *Yale Review* 9 (April, 1920): 452-61.

Kent, Frank. "Charley Michelson," *Scribner's Magazine* 188 (September, 1930): 290-96.

Knoll, Erwin. "The President and the Press: Eliminating the Middlemen," *Progressive* 34 (March, 1970): 13-18.

Krock, Arthur. "President Hoover's Two Years," *Current History* 34 (July, 1931): 488-94.

Lamont, Robert P. "The Personality of President Hoover," *Review of Reviews* 86 (September, 1932), 23-25.

Lippmann, Walter. "The Peculiar Weakness of Mr. Hoover," *Harper's Magazine* 161 (June, 1930): 1-7.

[Lorimer, George Horace]. "Demosthenes and Democracy" [Editorial], *Saturday Evening Post* 192 (November 15, 1919): 28-29.

Manning, George H. "Hoover Liberalizes Press Conferences: New Chief Executive Expected to Take Correspondents into Confidence," *Editor and Publisher* 61 (March 9, 1929): 7.

———. "'Tightening' of Press Relations Irks Washington Correspondents," *Editor and Publisher* 62 (July 6, 1929): 25.

————. "White House Is Best News Source for Rapidan Camp 100 Miles Away," *Editor and Publisher* 62 (July 13, 1929): 15.

McCann, Alfred W. "The Hoover Food-Control Failure," *Forum* 58 (October, 1917): 381-90.

Millis, Walter. "The President," *Atlantic Monthly* 149 (March, 1932): 265-78.

Moses, George. "The Misunderstood Hoover," *Liberty*, September, 1932.

"Political Notes: Presidential Prose," *Time* 26 (December 30, 1935): 8.

"The Presidency: The Hoover Week," *Time* 17 (April 27, 1931): 13.

Pringle, Henry F. "Hoover: An Enigma Easily Misunderstood," *World's Work* 56 (June, 1928): 131-43.

"Sacramento *Union* Is Sold by Allen," *Editor and Publisher* 54 (August 20, 1921): 37.

Shaw, A. W. "Simplification: A Philosophy of Business Management," *Harvard Business Review* 1 (June, 1923): 417-27.

————. "Startling Statements," *System* 40 (November, 1921): 534.

Stokes, Harold Phelps. "Smith and Hoover: A Comparison," *New York Times Magazine*, July 15, 1928, pp. 1-2, 22.

Strother, French. "Herbert Hoover: Representative American and Practical Idealist," *World's Work* 39 (April, 1920): 578-85.

Thurston, Elliott. "Hoover Can Not Be Elected," *Scribner's Magazine* 91 (January, 1932): 13-16.

Tucker, Ray T. "Is Hoover Human?" *North American Review* 226 (November, 1928): 513-19.

————. "Mr. Hoover Lays a Ghost," *North American Review* 227 (June, 1929): 661-69.

Wilhelm, Donald. "Bearding the Lions," *Independent* 99 (July 5, 1919): 21-23, 29.

————. "Hoover and His Food Organization," *Review of Reviews* 56 (September, 1917): 283-86.

————. "The Government's Own Publicity Work," *American Review of Reviews* 56 (November, 1917): 507-11.

————. "If He Were President: Herbert Hoover," *Independent* 100 (December 13, 1919): 170-71, 208, 210, 212-13.

————. "Mr. Hoover as Secretary of Commerce," *World's Work* 43 (February, 1922): 407-10.

————. "Waste Not, Want Not: An Interview with the United States Food Administrator," *Independent* 90 (June 9, 1917): 459-60.

———. "Working with Hoover: A Close-up View of a Great and Friendly Administrator," *World's Work* 56 (August, 1928): 410-16.

Index